May God ca

SOMETIMES

GOD SAYS

NO

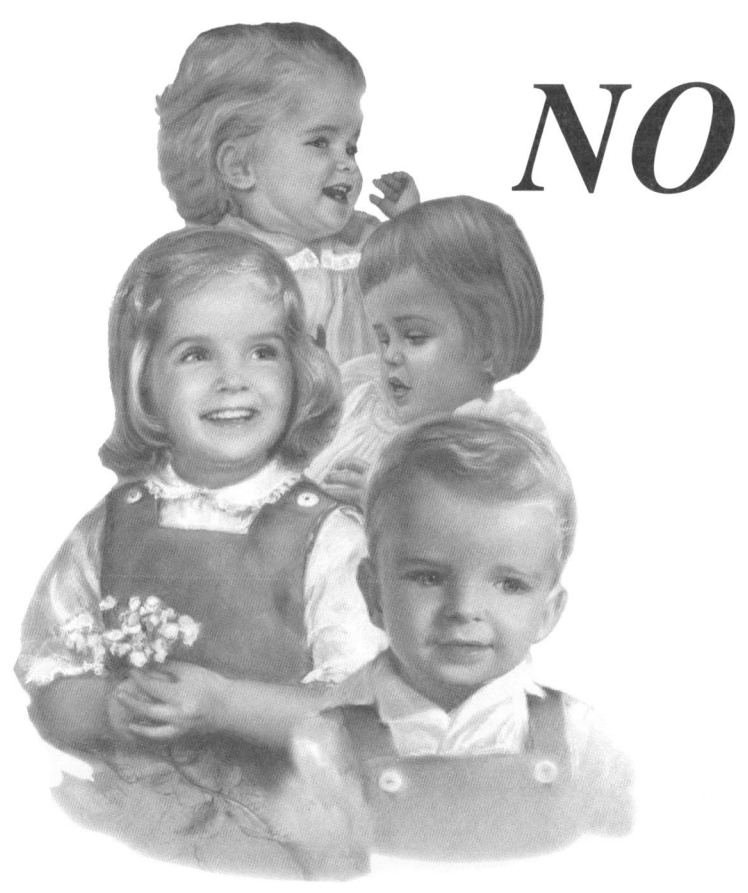

Ann Armstrong Peltier

Sometimes God Says No

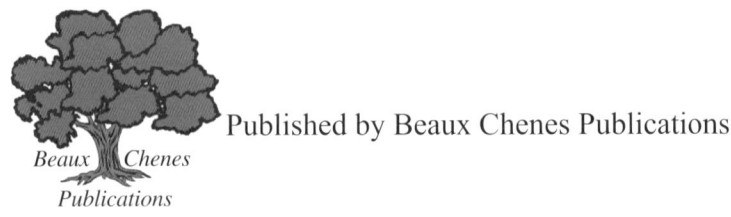 Published by Beaux Chenes Publications

Limited First Edition
Copyright © 2007 by Ann Armstrong Peltier

Unless otherwise identified, Bible quotations are from the New American Bible. Copyright © 1970, Confraternity of Christian Doctrine, Washington, D.C.

For information or to order copies of this book, contact:

Beaux Chenes Publications
567 Highway 308
Thibodaux, Louisiana 70301

ISBN: 978-0-9788770-0-2

The experiences noted in this autobiographical work are real. No slights of people or places are intentional.

Editing by Carol Pierce
Page layout by JANLO Services Publishing
Book/cover design by Carol Pierce and JANLO Services Publishing
Printed by MPress, New Orleans, LA 70125

Dedication

Sometimes God Says No is dedicated to my husband,

James Robert Peltier

Because he loved me and never let me down, I had courage, hope and patience. In his goodness, he came whenever I called and did his part.

Together we endured.

Table of Contents

Chapter One

Sometimes God Says No

$\mathcal{W}$hile attending a cocktail party with many of my good friends, I stood in a circle sipping my gin and tonic and listening to small talk. A newcomer chose to look at me and say, "What do you do?"

Why? I'll never know. I do know for a moment, I was speechless. I don't paint; I don't play tennis or golf; I don't do any of the interesting, creative things some in the circle can claim. I mumbled something about crocheting afghans, cooking and traveling.

Later, of course, I realized I could have said, "Over a period of fourteen years, I had four children with hydrocephalus. My husband and I consider those years our finest hours. None of these children ever knew the seriousness of their disease or realized they looked different from their peers. We never let them see us cry. I loved them completely, and I could feel them draw strength from me that sustained them and gave them courage during their times of pain."

Sometimes God Says No is an account of that fourteen-year period in my life when four of my children died from a rare condition called hydrocephalus. My husband and I also had one healthy child and adopted two boys from Ireland.

This story also talks about my conversion to the Roman Catholic religion – and my ensuing conflict with birth control.

It shows how my husband and I tried to live a normal life in spite of our children's illnesses and deaths, how our marriage was strengthened during these heartaches, and how my faith and love for God prevailed until the end.

Until now, those memories were far too dear to share with anyone. Each child enriched my life, and I selfishly wanted to keep all of them and those thoughts to myself.

Now I can think about our past. Now I realize my husband and I got up each morning and literally took up our cross and followed God.

At one time, that suffering was a daily routine for us, but now we are in a happy stretch of years. Had we not lived with those heartaches and crossed all those deep, depressing valleys, we may not today appreciate the health we have and the love we share. Just getting up, going to Mass, praying the Rosary, working, eating three meals a day, watching TV and being happy are a treasure. This normal life we now live free of illness is our Camelot.

I am sharing our story to help those of you in adversity and despair trust your faith and hold fast to hope. *Sometimes God Says No* is also for those of you bored with your ordinary lives. Perhaps you will be enriched by my memories and this story will help you value the treasure of a normal, healthy life.

I am also leaving this legacy to my daughter Jeanne, my wonderful healthy, normal daughter. If my husband and I could have written a prescription for what we would like in a daughter, we would have ordered Jeanne. She is the epitome of all our dreams.

I want our two adopted sons, Robert and David, to know we had courage when life was unbelievably discouraging, that we weren't afraid to take the risk of giving love again, and that we feel most fortunate to be the parents of two such fine young men.

Sometimes God Says No is also for my grandchildren so they can see the lives we lived.

I don't want this account to be depressing because our

lives weren't. We shared much joy and love; sadness was part of our happy life. Although ordinary words can't describe the heartaches and love we shared, ordinary words are all I have.

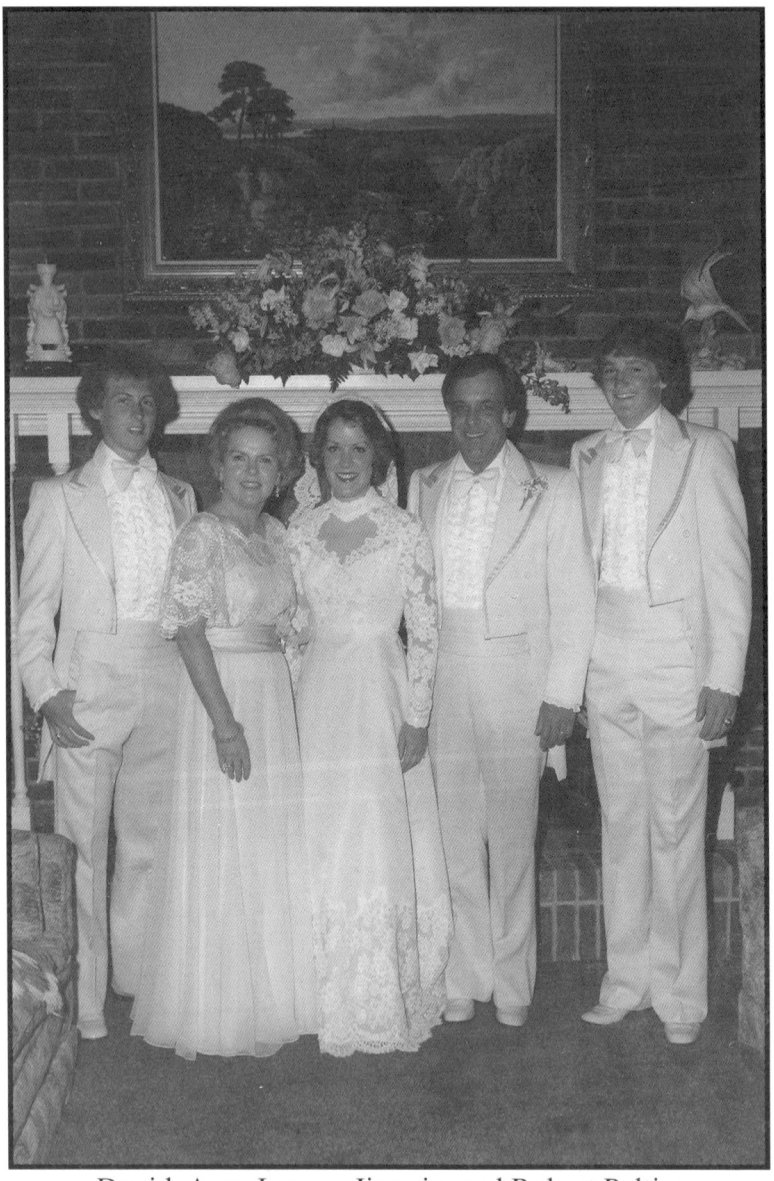

David, Ann, Jeanne, Jimmie, and Robert Peltier

Chapter Two

And So It Begins

$\mathcal{D}$own deep in the French part of Louisiana in that land of marshes and swamps, St. Joseph Cathedral stands tall and gaunt against the sky, its tall doors offering a welcome to those who come to the heart of the city of Thibodaux to worship God. Monsignor A. M. Barbier, the old French priest who designed and built this edifice in 1923, must have foreseen that worshipping God in such grand surroundings would enrich his parishioner's lives.

The Cathedral's interior is beautiful in the splendor of its sixteenth century French Renaissance architecture. The lovely rose window at the church's rear reminds me of the great one at Notre Dame in Paris. The gray, gold and blue ceilings, painted with lovely scenes depicting our Lord's life, are soothing and uplifting. I know this church well.

It was there the trumpets began to blare Mendelssohn's *Midsummer Night's Dream*… there my daughter Jeanne and her father began their long walk down the cathedral's aisle for her wedding.

Just a few minutes before, our two adopted sons had escorted me down the aisle to the front pew — Robert, very Irish looking, tall and slim with auburn hair; David, tall and trim with curly blonde hair. I felt proud to have them at my side, pleased to have my friends see these two impressive young men who are our sons. Most people knew the boys had come from Ireland to live with us shortly after their first birthdays. But Robert and David had spent their high school years away at boarding school, so many in the congregation were seeing them for the first time in years.

Amidst all the joy on that beautiful evening in June 1979, my thoughts drifted back to the four other important times I'd walked down that same aisle…the four times I had walked down the aisle of St. Joseph Cathedral to bury my children.

Our first child, Jim, was five years old when he died; Benita Ann was nine. Annette also lived to be nine, but Adrienne was only eight when we made that journey with her. A tombstone just a few blocks from the church attests to those four tragedies. Each time I see my four children's names and those dates etched into the black marble, I still find it hard to believe what happened to Jimmie and me.

All four children—Jim, Benita Ann, Annette, and Adrienne—died from a rare condition called hydrocephalus. The name means water (hydro) in the head (cephale). The condition is characterized by an abnormal increase in the amount of fluid in the cranium, causing the head to enlarge, the brain to waste away, and mental powers to be lost.

When we first learned the diagnosis for our son Jim, doctors told us that only one child in a thousand has hydrocephalus. That news was hard enough to accept at the time. It's even harder now to believe we had four children with this tragic condition. I had seven pregnancies. Two ended in miscarriages; one child was normal; four had hydrocephalus.

*****

I grew up in a small southern Louisiana town. Like all good Baptists, my parents took me to all the church services. There was Sunday school class at 9:45 a.m., the church service at 10:45 a.m. and Baptist Training Union at 7:30 p.m. On Wednesday evenings we went to service, also. Sometimes when the revivals came to town, we attended church under a tent with a sawdust floor.

When I was five, I remember walking down a long, sawdust aisle to the front of the revival tent to recite the Twenty-Third Psalm. Afterwards, the Preacher gave me a nickel.

I truly felt the Lord was my shepherd. I loved God with all my heart and soul. My youth ran smoothly through green pastures, and I gave God credit. My prayers, although undemanding, had always been answered. I believed God would provide the man who'd become my special Prince Charming when the right time came. And He did.

My life was a sheltered one at a time when stamps for letters to the outside world cost only three cents. When we moved from the small Louisiana town of Montgomery to another named DeRidder, my mother became concerned for my safety. Because of World War II, many soldiers were at nearby Fort Polk. I had many warnings to be careful. High school was football, jitterbugging at school dances, and swimming parties at Bundix Creek. DeRidder was dry, but we never really noticed. We were intoxicated with life.

Chemistry was my best subject, and, on the advice of my high school counselor, I entered Louisiana State University in the fall of 1947 to major in Hospital Dietetics. I left DeRidder for the large college town of Baton Rouge and a new life full of enthusiasm and apprehension.

Sororities were very important to every girl from DeRidder attending LSU. Although rush week was a harrowing experience, I survived and very happily pledged Chi Omega. The friends and security I found at LSU helped me become more involved in campus activities. Mortar Board, Phi Kappa Phi, outstanding senior in the College of Agriculture. My life was different, but the pastures remained green, and the waters still. Everything went well.

In 1951, I interned at Charity Hospital in New Orleans after graduating from LSU. Jimmie Peltier was in his sophomore year at Loyola University Dental School in New Orleans. Although we had seen each other from a distance on the LSU

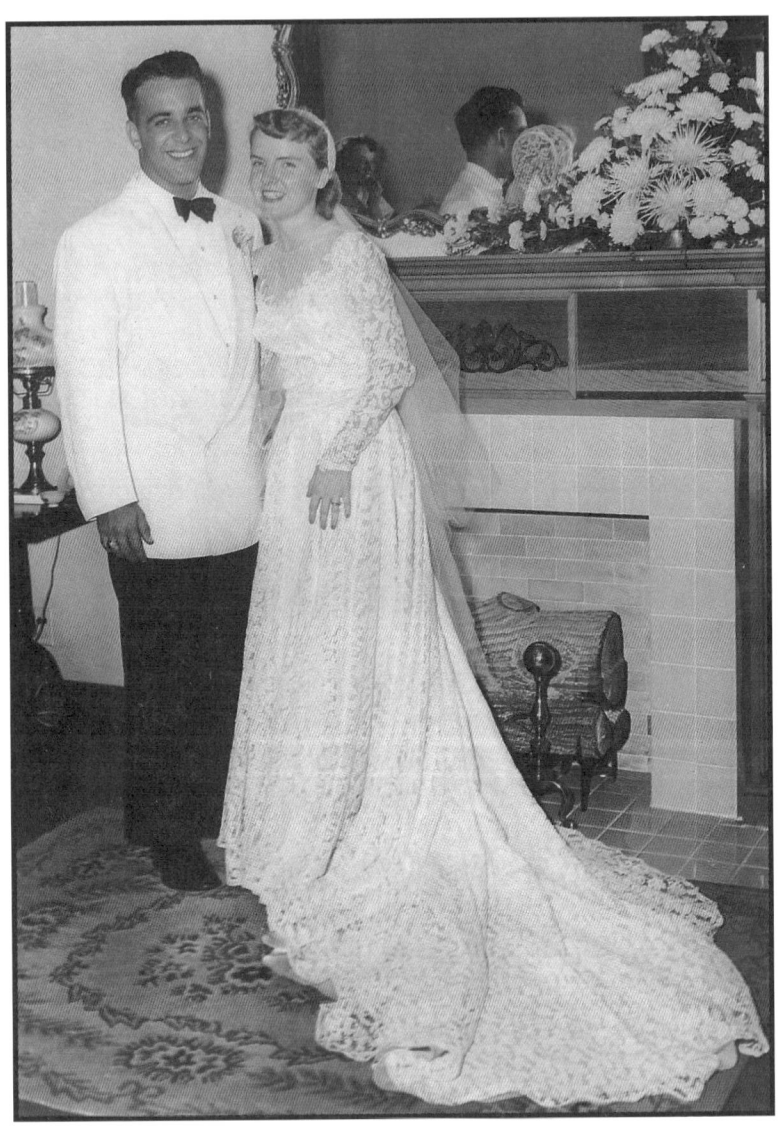

Dr. and Mrs. James Robert Peltier

campus, we had never actually talked until we met at a Dental School dance. I had a blind date; Jimmie asked me to dance. A guest at his table told me later that upon returning to his chair, Jimmie said, "I just danced with the girl I'm going to marry." My Prince Charming had found me.

Jimmie and I had an exciting time before we married. We saw New Orleans together. We went to LSU football games. We even went to the fights at the Civic Center. I loved being in his presence. I loved watching him walk toward me when he came to pick me up. I found him exciting.

But the biggest problem during our courtship was that he was a Roman Catholic and I a Baptist. After our having many of what we, at twenty years of age, thought were intelligent, well-thought-out talks on the subject, we decided that, basically, we both believed in God. Because of this common belief, we felt we could overcome our religious differences, so we set our wedding date.

On August 10, 1952, I became Mrs. James Robert Peltier. Because ours was a mixed marriage, we weren't allowed to be married at the altar of the small wooden St. Joseph Church in DeRidder. However, we were allowed to have music and flowers, which meant a lot to me. Our families accepted our mixed marriage. They were very supportive, and we were happy.

In January 1953, after six months of marriage, I awakened in the night with terrible abdominal pains. I knew I was four months pregnant, but I never dreamed what was happening to me at that moment was a miscarriage. Just that day a pregnant friend had told me to expect pain during pregnancy. For a long time, I tried to ignore what I was feeling, but the pain finally became so severe I had to awaken Jimmie.

How young we were. How little we knew. We had no doctor to call because we planned to return to Jimmie's hometown of Thibodaux for our baby's birth, and I had been seeing a gynecologist there.

Instead of going to an emergency room, we called Dr.

Richard Morvant, an old friend who was completing his surgical residency at Charity Hospital. By the time Dickie got to our apartment, it was too late to move me to a hospital. He made me as comfortable as possible through that dark, painful night while I suffered a miscarriage. Dickie baptized the baby, and Jimmie and I had our first angel in Heaven.

Dr. T. Benton "Ben" Ayo, my gynecologist in Thibodaux, subsequently consoled me by saying, "Ann, very often a female body will reject an imperfect fetus."

At that time, I brushed away the idea. Jimmie and I were young and in love. We surely would have other children. We had ahead of us our whole life together. Jimmie was a junior in Dental School and felt confident he could complete the curriculum. While he rode the streetcar to Loyola each day, I took my household duties very seriously. I cooked, cleaned house, read, and in my free time, played a little bridge.

Because Jimmie was having dental clinical practical experience, his evenings were usually free, so 1953 became a time of our dashing to the movies. There were so many good movies that we would run across Canal Street from the Saenger Theatre to the Loew's State Theatre to see two movies a night. We had such good times. Once we carved meat on our new silver wedding-present trays, making large dents in them. I still enjoy looking at those dented silver trays, reminders of how young and happy we were.

During that time, Jimmie went to the Catholic services on Sundays and holy days of obligation. I continued to attend the Baptist Church. Although we attended some services with each other in our respective places of worship, I was aware of how much Jimmie wanted me to study Catholicism. After a time, I admitted I would like to have a better understanding of his religion.

Jimmie knew Father Thomas Atherton, a Jesuit priest Jimmie felt would be a good teacher for me. So I went to Loyola at prescribed times to study with Father Atherton. Because Jimmie and I were fortunate enough to have one of the first television sets and boxing matches were at their peak of popularity, Father Atherton often promoted the idea of his coming to our old New Orleans style apartment on Joseph Street to give me a lesson. Those lessons often adjourned early so he could watch the boxing matches. We had such a good time!

I liked studying about the Catholic Church. Much to my surprise, the discussions I thought would be undemanding began to challenge my thinking. The books I thought I'd casually read made me take a closer look at myself and life. I began to see and love God in a deeper, more meaningful way. Those studies opened up another dimension of my worship to Him. Something I'd begun in order to understand Jimmie's religion better was enriching my mind and changing my values.

The aspect of Catholicism I liked best was transubstantiation, the heart of the Mass when the bread and wine is actually changed into God's body and blood. I liked reliving the last supper each time I was at Mass, knowing this was a sacrifice just as in the Old Testament when Abraham made sacrifices to God. I liked the idea that daily services were available for me to worship God. I liked the privacy attending Mass offered me and the idea that I worshipped God with dignity. I liked the meaning of Catholic – that the Mass was the same all over the world.

Confession was at first difficult to accept, but before I fell asleep each night as a child, I recalled the sins committed that day and would ask God to forgive them. As a Catholic, I could do the same, but with the extra promise that God gave to his priests, "Whose sins you forgive are forgiven, and whose sins you retain shall be retained."

Although the disappointment my family would feel if I became a Catholic weighed on me, I knew I had to become a Catholic to partake of the body and blood of Christ after I read John 6: 48-58 in the Bible. In this chapter, John reminds us that Jesus said to them, "Amen, amen, I say to you, unless you eat the flesh of the Son of Man and drink his blood, you do not have life within you. Whoever eats my flesh and drinks my blood has eternal life, and I will raise him on the last day."

I knew how very trying Jimmie and I marrying in a Catholic ceremony in 1952 was for my mother. He and I were required to sign papers in which I promised to rear my children as Catholics and to never interfere with Jimmie's practice of his religion. Once again, I saw the love my mother had for me when she witnessed my signing those papers. I know how painful it was for her.

As we would lay awake at night, Jimmie taught me Catholic prayers – the *Hail Mary, I Believe in God, Prayer for Faith, Hope and Charity*, and the morning and evening prayers.

After over a year of studying with Father Atherton, I announced I'd like to become a Catholic. Both he and Jimmie said, "No, you need to learn more. You must be absolutely sure."

Because my hometown of DeRidder was largely Protestant, Jimmie and Father Atherton wanted me to be certain that if I ever went back to DeRidder, I could live happily in the Catholic Church. Their response surprised me, but it spurred me to do more reading and thinking as I continued my studies with Father Atherton.

On July 26, 1953, I was baptized in the Holy Name of Jesus Church on stately old St. Charles Avenue in New Orleans. I'd been baptized as a child in the Baptist Church, but the Catholic Church required that these rites be performed again. Jimmie's mother was my sponsor, and I began my life as a Catholic with a deep abiding faith and thankfulness. God had given me a chance to worship Him in what I considered a more meaningful way.

Because the baptismal rite, my first confession, and my first communion were very important to me, I thought I'd experience a special feeling or some special way of knowing God was pleased. Father Atherton hastened to tell me there is no sign, no extraordinary wave of feeling that sweeps one away when receiving the sacraments. One has to know mentally that the soul is receiving grace.

One of the hardest church teachings for me to understand was about indulgences. An indulgence is the remission in whole or part of the temporal punishment due to sin. There are two types. A plenary indulgence is the full remission of the temporal punishment due to sin. A partial indulgence is the remission of a part of that temporal punishment.

Grasping the meaning and being thankful for this gift the church offers, I decided to devote my life to gaining plenary indulgences for the souls in Purgatory. But to gain these indulgences, I must be in a state of grace, having just gone to confession within eight days of also attending Mass, receiving communion, and praying for the Pope. I marvel at this powerful gift the Catholic Church offers its members.

If I had to sum up why I wanted to become a Catholic, I would say it is because I saw the Mass as the best way for me to worship God – the best way to show my love for Him. I also liked being able to attend Mass alone. I could go anytime anywhere and have no one notice me. I liked this private touch with God. Being a Catholic has enriched my life, and I am thankful now I made that decision. It has been a mainstay for me through all of my children's illnesses and their ensuing deaths.

The first summer after Jimmie and I were married, we visited Washington, New York, and Canada. The highlight of our trip was our visit to the shrine honoring the Blessed Mother's mother. High in the mountains of Canada out from Montreal is the magnificent church of St. Anne de Beaupre. Jimmie and I saw the walls of crutches discarded by cripples suddenly able to walk again. Our visit to this place of miracles was a moving experience for us both. Where so many others had prayed with deep piety, we prayed for a baby. I will always remember those prayers.

In August we found that we were "that way" again. What a great few months we had. My cup was running over.

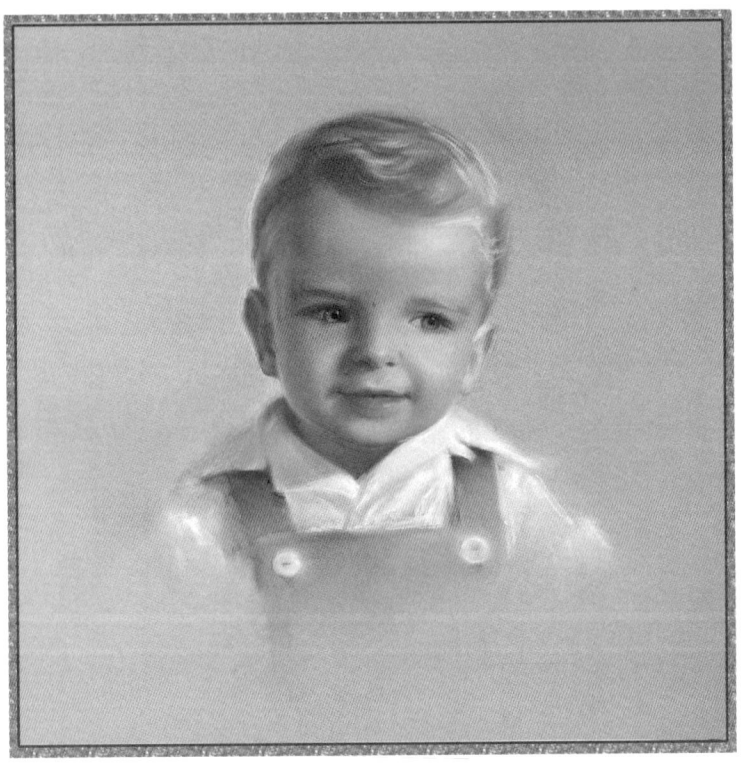

James Robert Peltier, Jr.

Chapter Three

Our First Child, Jim

*O*n April 8, 1954, we had our son. He was born six weeks early. This time when the labor pains started, we rushed to the hospital. His birth went smoothly, and when I awakened, my mother, as always, was once again there when I needed her.

How wonderful to have a son to name after my husband — James Robert Peltier, Jr. We decided we'd call our baby Jim. Jim had always been a name I associated with a big, blustering truck driver, but now Jim meant a gorgeous little blonde boy I adored.

Since Jim weighed less than five pounds at birth, he had to stay in the hospital for a time after I was discharged. One day I stood outside the viewing window looking at Jim and wishing I could hold him. A large black man weighing nearly three hundred pounds was sweeping the floor. He stopped, looked at Jim, and said, "Don't worry, ma'am. I didn't weigh but two and a half pounds, and look at me now."

Five weeks after his birth, we placed our newborn into a bassinette covered in blue eyelet and ribbon. With love and care, we happily settled Jim into our life at 1445 Joseph Street.

Finally, the day for Jimmie's graduation from Loyola Dental School arrived. As I was changing Jim's diaper, he urinated in a perfect stream into Jimmie's mortarboard. That night at graduation, I felt sure Jimmie was the only person on

15

stage receiving a doctorate degree while wearing a wet hat. We still laugh when we remember that incident.

Following his graduation, Jimmie was inducted into the United States Air Force. His orders read, "Patrick Air Force Base, Cocoa Beach, Florida, to be preceded by three weeks of basic training at Gunter Air Force Base, Alabama."

Before leaving for duty, we'd divide the summer between Jimmie's hometown and mine. First, we'd drive to Thibodaux to spend a few days, then we would go to DeRidder so I could show off my beautiful baby boy. Other friends also had new babies, so we were all eager to meet and share our new treasures.

Jimmie and I decided that spending a few days at Grand Isle between these two family visits would be relaxing. Grand Isle is a barrier island off the Louisiana coast where Jimmie spent all of his childhood summers fishing, swimming, and playing in the sun. Because mosquitoes were so bad that year, everyone felt Jim would be better off staying in Thibodaux. We agreed. A trusted friend offered to keep him, so Jimmie and I departed happily.

When we returned two days later, I noticed a subtle change in Jim. He was still handsome, but his head appeared larger. When a change is so slight, it is hard to convince anyone a problem exists, particularly when no one wants to be convinced.

During my internship as a dietician at Charity Hospital, I had seen the hydrocephalic ward. It was tucked in the back of the hospital where few people visited unless they had a particular reason for doing so. Why I had been drawn to that ward, I don't know, but I had visited it many times. It was such a heartbreaking place.

The beds were filled with children with enormous heads. I didn't know their history, nor did I know why modern surgery had allowed their heads to become so enlarged. The protruding veins on their large heads, looking like large lines on a map, made a horrible sight even worse. Parents had abandoned most of these children.

Remembering that ward at Charity Hospital, I had the horrible thought Jim might have the same condition. I took some comfort from Jimmie's family, who assured me they could see no change in our baby's looks. Surely I was imagining it. Even in my anxiety that Jim might have this same disfiguring condition, I didn't begin to realize the horror of it all.

Finally, I talked Jimmie into letting me telephone our old friend Dr. Morvant about my concerns. By this time, Dickie had completed his surgery residency and was practicing in Thibodaux.

I told Dr. Morvant, "Dickie, maybe he has hydrocephalus."

I remember well his reply, "Of course, he doesn't have that! Hydrocephalus is rare!"

I'm sure he thought, *Another young, anxious mother with a terrific imagination.*

"However," he said, "a pediatrician has just moved into the area to practice in Raceland. Just to put your mind at ease, I'll get an appointment for you tomorrow morning."

That fifteen-mile trip to Raceland was long. Jimmie was trying to look so in charge when down deep inside he was really frightened. I was holding Jim and thinking, *This is not happening!* I even said, "Jimmie, I don't know a thing about hydrocephalus except what I saw at Charity. From what I remember, those children live to be only about eight years old."

In that dark, depressing building that was still under construction, the young pediatrician seeing his first patient made one exploratory touch of the fontanel and told us Jim had hydrocephalus.

Jimmie and I sat there completely stunned, trying to be intelligent, straight-thinking parents while the doctor explained hydrocephalus to us. He told us it was, indeed, rare and that he knew a neurosurgeon in New Orleans making great strides in surgery for this condition.

I'm sure that pediatrician was happy to see us leave and relieved to be rid of the responsibility as he watched us walk away, knowing what lay ahead of us.

As I look back, I thank God for my youth, my faith, and my love for Jimmie. I felt driven to try to keep Jimmie's spirits up. By seeing him stern, accepting, and hopeful, I could have hope.

Jimmie and I returned to Thibodaux and sought Dickie's advice. Dickie called to make an appointment with the neurosurgeon, Dr. José Garcia Oller, a man who would be a part of our lives for a long time to come.

Our original visit to Dr. Garcia is a hazy memory. We sat very still as we listened to Dr. Garcia explain Jim's possible condition. Hydrocephalus is rare, occurring in approximately one in every thousand births. The condition can be congenital or can result from an infection, a brain tumor, an injury, or other less frequent causes. The term is applied to any condition in which the ventricular system enlarges. The ventricles are the cavities inside the brain containing cerebrospinal fluid. When there is an imbalance between the fluid produced and that absorbed, hydrocephalus results.

Obstructive hydrocephalus occurs when a blockage prevents that fluid from flowing out of the ventricles into the space between the two layers of the brain. Because the cerebrospinal fluid can't leave the ventricles, fluid pressure builds and causes the ventricles to expand, the outer brain to thin and the person's head to enlarge. That blockage point in the brain is technically known as the Aqueduct of Sylvias. It is a tiny pathway no larger than the diameter of a pine needle. Four of our children developed congenital obstructive hydrocephalus.

Because Jim was already six weeks old, Dr. Garcia felt surgery should be done soon to eliminate that increased pressure. The size of Jim's head had increased somewhat but was not terribly large.

I have learned doctors don't reveal everything at once. I suppose they reason that each step is a new surprise and that there are two possible results from any treatment — good or bad. If the results are good, why should the patient know the alternative? If results are bad, then there is time to readjust.

Unfortunately, our experiences seemed to all too frequently end with a bad result. Each step was a new and rarely pleasant surprise, yet Jimmie and I clung together to keep each other's spirits up, adjusting day after day.

At twenty-two years of age, we seemed caught up in some impossible web that felt like a vise closing in around us. Family and friends tried their best to help, tried to say the right words because they loved us. But what can one say to parents of a beautiful first-born son with such a deforming condition?

One of my worse problems was my knowing how much this hurt Jimmie — his having a man's dream, a son, and for that son to have such a terrible affliction. I resolved to try my best to help Jimmie and to try to always be hopeful.

Jimmie must have made the same resolution because he stood by me always. Just seeing him gave me strength. When his eyes met mine, I knew we had the same thoughts. We reached an unspoken agreement that no matter what was happening inside our child's body, no matter what horrors lay ahead, we'd try to keep our baby happy, try to think happy thoughts, and tomorrow and the next day and the day after that, we'd do the same. We were all three in this together. Each of us would play the roles assigned us the very best we could in order to give the other two courage.

Having had children of my own, I now know what parents suffer when their child suffers. I had been an only child. My father had been ill most of his adult life. During my very early years, my mother went through the agony of accepting his illness without any support or comfort from his family. Alone, she had to convince officials of the overcrowded Veterans Administration Hospital that he was sick and needed to be admitted. That was in the 1930's, the Great Depression years. Money was scarce, and she had to work to support us.

Because Mother did a marvelous job of keeping Dad's illness and her anxieties from me, I have very few unpleasant memories of those days. She was a tower of strength. I never saw her shed any tears in public, but I am certain many were shed when she was alone. She always gave me love and a sense of security when I needed them as a child and as a woman. Her strong love gave me courage and strength. No matter what I did or how I did it, she accepted me unconditionally. One of the sustaining forces through my children's illnesses was the certainty that my mother was always there, always ready to talk when I called.

I was nervous about making that first call to tell my mother about Jim's illness, but I decided I would tell her the truth rather than hide some facts. If she could closely follow each step, maybe the events would be easier to take. I really didn't want her to suffer these heartaches and wished this problem could be mine and Jimmie's alone. But when a mother's love is involved, a couple's problems don't belong just to them. When I made that call, my mom once again said all the right things to me.

Next, we called Jimmie's family. Jimmie is one of five children. Each person in his family did everything humanly possible to make our trials easier to bear. They came. They came in numbers. They sat patiently waiting with us. They took us individually out to eat so one of us could always be at the hospital with Jim. When people of French origin get together, there is always conversation. During those family visits, those conversations diverted our thoughts for moments at a time.

However, I really felt badly about interrupting everyone's lives. They all had large families back at home as well as important jobs; I was well aware of the sacrifices they were making and loved them for it.

*****

On June 25, 1954, Jimmie and I brought Jim to Mercy Hospital in New Orleans for the very first time. Dr. Garcia explained about the fontanel on our baby's head (sometimes called the soft spot) and what it meant. Since fluid couldn't drain from Jim's head, his soft spot was bulging. The bones of his skull, which were soft at his age, were expanding to allow room for his fluid-enlarged brain. However, if an over-abundance of fluid would build, the pressure increase inside his brain could cause projectile vomiting and lead to brain damage, as well as disfigurement.

Dr. Garcia wanted to know if Jim had experienced those symptoms. He hadn't. Because Jim's pupils would be forced downward, his eyes would be an indication of an increase in pressure. Dr. Garcia also added that excess pressure could cause convulsions that could lead to a coma.

In some cases, when these symptoms become acute, it's necessary to remove fluid or tap a child's head with a large needle to relieve the pressure. This aspiration has to be done with extreme care to prevent too much fluid removal at one time or too quickly to prevent the brain from collapsing. That would cause death.

Subtly, Dr. Garcia revealed that occasionally a tap or two causes the blockage to open. He'd seen some babies cured as well as partial blockages correct themselves. We were somewhat encouraged when Dr. Garcia mentioned some great men in history had been hydrocephalic for a time in their infancy. We listened.

Dr. Garcia ordered major tests to rule out a possible brain tumor and to determine the exact type of hydrocephalus affecting Jim. One of the tests was a pneumoencephalogram. In this procedure, a bubble of air would be injected into Jim's brain. A series of x-rays would then be taken to follow the air bubble while Jim would be in different positions. This test would determine where the fluid flow blockage was and would help diagnose a possible brain tumor.

When the time for this testing procedure arrived, I was holding Jim in my arms in the hall outside of the Radiology Examination Room. When the door opened and Dr. Garcia reached for Jim, I handed my baby to him. Doing so marked my first surrender. Suddenly, I thought about the Blessed Mother as she handed Jesus to Simeon at the Presentation. Desperately, I tried to trust God with all of my heart as His Mother trusted Him.

After reviewing the results of Jim's tests, Dr. Garcia told us Jim had a complete blockage. Dr. Garcia would have to surgically shunt the excess fluid by bypassing this blockage. To accomplish this, a plastic tube would be placed from Jim's ventricle, where the fluid was accumulating, to a reservoir in his neck. The fluid could then be distributed normally to Jim's body. This operation, known as the Torkildson procedure, is the most natural of all the possible surgical procedures.

Dr. Garcia favored using this procedure at the time because Jim's head wouldn't grow as rapidly at this age as his torso. If the disease could be arrested without affecting Jim's torso, the results would be more normal and advantageous. Dr. Garcia also told us that with this procedure, Jim's tube wouldn't need changing as quickly as with other available options. Without surgery, Jim would live for approximately three months.

Jimmie and I were at Dr. Garcia's complete mercy and were anxious to proceed with the surgery in order to stop the daily, almost hourly, enlargement of Jim's head. Of course, we had every hope the operation would succeed.

We found ourselves staring at Dr. Garcia's hands. I still remember those small hands with long, thin fingers and prominent knuckles. These were certainly, we thought, the kind of hands a neurosurgeon ought to have.

I kept praying God would guide Dr. Garcia in what seemed an insurmountable task – curing our child.

Chapter Four

First Surgery

$\mathcal{T}$he day for Jim's surgery arrived. The operation under local anesthesia lasted eight hours. That day was interminable, and all seemed so impossible.

When Jim was given the pneumoencephalogram and the dye test, I had the first hint of the feelings I'd experience while he was in surgery. Over and over, I'd experience those feelings as I sat waiting while someone I loved had his body strangely altered by surgery or endured treatments that caused pain. To sit quietly, properly dressed, and looking normal seemed strange when on the inside, I felt a horror that can only be compared to a nightmare. I realized such events were out of my control completely. I'd have to wait for things to take their course. If there had been somewhere to run for protection as I used to run to my mother's consoling arms as a child, I'd probably have run.

But now as an adult, running wasn't a choice. I had to sit quietly. I had to turn everything over to God. I found it hard to submit to God and difficult to say "Thy will be done" as I tried to analyze what He wanted most of me. I knew He'd want me to be near my child and turn full control over to Him, so I tried to fulfill His wish.

When Dr. Garcia walked into the waiting room eight hours later, he looked surprisingly fresh after such a long, tiring procedure. He said, "Well, we did what we set out to do."

I lived to learn that those words were the most important statement a surgeon could make. Being so young, I couldn't have foreseen all that could have gone wrong and could have prevented the surgery from being completed. Later I learned to listen for that statement first. "We did what we set out to do" meant everything.

Private duty nurses were ordered because of the seriousness of the surgery and the special care Jim needed, but Jimmie and I were always there.

The doctor felt it best Jim wear only a diaper since he was running fever. Obviously, the necessary drainage was taking place. Strict orders were given to roll him from side to side frequently. Because the surgical incision ran down the back of his neck, he had to be left in bed alone without being held although my arms ached to hold him.

Jim loved his pacifier. Alone on cold sheets in a bed without being held, he could at least find comfort sucking on his pacifier as he cooed, kicked and played with the suspended toys. Jim was beautiful, and by now, he was an adorable age.

Just walking into Jim's hospital room and seeing him gave me great joy. One of the unexplained side effects of the accumulating fluid is it can stimulate the brain. Sometimes the patient is brighter because of this pressure. I didn't consider this at the time, but Jim was extremely alert after his surgery, responding to us with smiles and kicks. I can still see his well-formed, naturally tan little body, with his legs kicking and arms waving in the air. Jim's room at Mercy Hospital was a happy room.

What amazed me most was we all still appeared normal. We made small conversation, smiled, and read the paper. I don't know what I expected us to do. In spite of the overpowering inner turmoil, we continued to live. In the face of Jim's hydrocephalus, we still had hope and stamina to overcome our adversities. If we hadn't had hope along the way, we couldn't have persevered.

Earlier I spoke of the close relationship I've had with God all my life. He always answered my prayers, so I thought He would once again answer them. I was so naïve that I didn't realize there was a possibility He wouldn't cure Jim.

Jimmie and I spent many hours kneeling in the small chapel tucked away at the end of a hall off the first floor of Mercy Hospital. Kneeling in the dark shadows when the chapel was not in use, we prayed, beseeching God to help us. We tried earnestly to pray, "Thy will be done." But into our prayers always crept, "Let the shunt work; let the shunt drain Jim's head; please let us go home with our baby."

From everywhere came religious medals and prayers written in elaborate calligraphy. Dozens of medals were pinned or tied to Jim's bed with colorful ribbons – medals that had brought miraculous cures to so many people. These medals and ribbons always made me feel strange because I wasn't accustomed to this particular way of interceding with God. There was no religious article such as this in the Baptist Church I had known as a child.

And yet, we felt everyone, Baptist and Catholic alike in both our hometowns, was praying for us. People were so good! Orders of nuns called and wrote, offering their special contact with God for us, and priests came to give their blessings. With each piece of encouragement, we just knew we could triumph over this, that God would surely answer so many heartfelt prayers.

Then Jimmie and I began to notice Jim's fontanel wasn't always sunken. Some days it was more full than others. It became so firm the doctor thought Jim's head should be tapped. This procedure sounded horrible, but we were assured it wasn't painful because the brain itself has no nerve endings that elicit pain. The doctors could slip the needle in to aspirate the fluid without causing much discomfort to Jim. In fact, the doctors told us Jim even looked around and smiled as the pressure lessened. The dramatic change in Jim after the tap was hard to believe. Moments before, he had been cross and irritable.

After the tap, he was as lively as could be.

Time in the hospital dragged on with no end in sight as days began to turn into weeks. Dr. Garcia admitted another baby with hydrocephalus. John was placed across the hall from Jim. His parents had that desperate look we came to know all too well from parents with sick children.

During the long hours of each day, hours that seemed endless because of our concern for our babies, Jim and I and Sugar and John Morrison, John's parents, became close friends. We shared the same problems, and each of us could find some solace in discussing our confused thoughts.

We each had come from a small town, and our only previous contact with the medical profession had been with doctors who were friends of the family. Those doctors had shown concern and love when we were sick.

Because of that, it took all of us time to adjust to Dr. Garcia's manner of relating to his patients. He smiled and was always solicitous, yet distant and aloof. He exuded confidence, but he remained apart from the patient and his family. Even as the months dragged on and he knew us better, there was no change in his attitude. We began to learn from his conversations that he was an extremely religious man. However, we were always conscious that he was the doctor and we were the dependent parents of the patient.

There were so many new things to learn in this new situation that it was easy to become overwhelmed and confused. Jimmie and I were able to talk with the Morrisons about Dr. Garcia to try to understand why he remained so aloof. Finally, the four of us decided because he was a neurosurgeon and all of his patients were desperately ill, he couldn't allow himself to become emotionally involved with his patients or their families. Talking to Sugar and John helped me a great deal in feeling more comfortable around Dr. Garcia.

Their little John didn't have the alertness and stamina Jim had. Yet his surgery was performed, and the shunt seemed to work immediately. He was in the hospital for a little over three weeks and went home while we stayed on as we sadly found out all shunts work differently from child to child. With occasional taps, Jim was better, but in a few days, his fontanel was bulging again, and he needed another tap. It began to dawn on us that we weren't going to leave the hospital as soon as we had hoped after all.

Before we knew Jim had hydrocephalus and right after Jimmie's graduation from dental school in 1954, the Air Force had moved all our household goods to Cocoa Beach, Florida. July was fast approaching; Jimmie had to report for active duty. He would go first to Gunter Air Force Base for three weeks basic training and then to Patrick Air Force Base in Florida.

When Jim was admitted into Mercy Hospital for his surgery, Jimmie and I rented an apartment in New Orleans to use for bathing and what little sleep we could manage between our times at the hospital with Jim. We had been renting this apartment for two months when family and friends in New Orleans invited me to stay with them in their homes while Jimmie entered the service of his country. I gladly accepted their invitation.

Here was my husband, Jimmie, ordered by the U.S. Government to report for service. At the same time, here lay our child who couldn't leave the hospital because at any moment, he might need a tap to relieve him of increased fluid pressure. My prayers now took on a new dimension. "Please, God, show me what to do, and give me the courage to carry it through."

I began to learn that to get through this hard time, I would have to take one day at a time and forget what I wanted to happen. I learned to be cheerful even when I didn't feel that way. Before, I always had some control over my life. I could make plans for the future and go wherever I wanted. Now, I didn't really know what might happen the next day or the next month. And I had to be wherever our son Jim was.

The day came when Jimmie had to leave. I wanted so badly

to go with him. It was a struggle to stay; yet as I watched him, I knew he found it worse to go. Here he was — a man with a wife and a baby, a very sick baby, he had to leave behind to go to an unknown world he'd have to face alone, knowing no one there.

The empty house waiting for Jimmie with all our newly acquired belongings only emphasized his grief. In the service, one's time is not his own. Jimmie was no longer his own boss. Just losing that freedom was a difficult adjustment for him. Literally, it was a time of growing up for both of us, and we each drew strength from deep down within ourselves. There were no tears. We didn't need to discuss our inner struggles. We each had to meet this new phase in our life in our own way.

After Jimmie left, I thought my world would end. Much to my surprise, I lived on as always; I bathed and dressed the best way I could; and I ate three meals a day. The best part of all was I found immense joy with my little boy. I loved being in Jim's presence, spending every minute with him. With that marvelous invention of Alexander Graham Bell, Jimmie and I shared each day and gave each day meaning in spite of how we really felt torn apart.

There were the hours we spent praying. Jimmie went to Mass whenever possible, and I attended services in New Orleans. Jimmie wrote me every day. When the mailman delivered several letters, those were happy times. Jimmie's letters made me think and gave me a much deeper understanding of this man I had married and loved with all my heart.

August 16, 1954: Edward's (a cousin of Jimmie's ordained in Belgium as a Jesuit priest) ordination – "I hope he remembers our baby in his first Mass."

August 14, 1954: "I finished the book, *The Woman Shall Conquer*, and it really is good. It helps in the devotion to Mary."

August 23, 1954: "If we suffer for a purpose and with God in mind, it cannot help but be pleasing in Heaven. If you look at it like that, we have a wonderful opportunity to suffer for

Him. It is soothing to think of getting something out of Jim's illness anyway."

September 16, 1954: "Hope James, Jr. is still doing well, but let me know if anything happens. You know I think of Jim differently these last six weeks, i.e., of him being well fairly soon, which is a much different light than before. Now it's mostly heartache between you and me. But it's too bad most people cannot get a good scare like we did to see what they are on this earth for. I guess some get it, but don't see it. Anyway, I'm glad I got so much out of this."

September 21, 1954: "But, remember, all this suffering won't go for naught. It's being registered in that book up there – time off in Purgatory."

Once Jimmie had completed his three weeks of basic training in Alabama, I traveled by train to meet him there and to drive with him to Florida to set up housekeeping. Being together again for a few days gave us some respite. Although leaving Jimmie in strange and new surroundings was very difficult, I knew my place was back at the hospital with our son.

The long days and nights I spent alone at the hospital gave me time to read and think. I began exploring the lives of the saints. St. Theresa, The Little Flower, was one of my favorites. I cherished the story of her falling from the pony, looking up and saying to God, "If this is how you treat those who love you, no wonder you have so few friends."

Learning about the human side of these favorites of God made me search for even more literature. I learned about St. Rita, a mystic who suffered the crown of thorns around her head; St. Theresa of Avila, who founded a new religious order so many years ago in Avila, Spain; St. Ignatius Loyola from Barcelona, Spain, who founded the Society of Jesus, the Jesuit order to which Father Atherton belonged.

Novenas were something I'd never heard of as a member of the Baptist Church, so they were a wonderful new experience. A novena is a nine-day public or private devotion that can be said to obtain special graces. Since some of those novenas are known to never fail, I set about making all sorts of nine-day requests for Jim.

Whenever I could, I'd visit various churches to pray to that particular saint. New Orleans has many churches, each named after a different saint. I visited the churches near Mercy Hospital first, one of which is the Sacred Heart of Jesus Church on Canal Street. Next, I visited the churches dedicated to St. Ann and St. Jude. I even explored the grottos on the church grounds whenever possible. I was especially fond of St. Joseph Church on Tulane Avenue. I had walked by that church many times during my training to become a dietitian at Charity Hospital, never realizing someday I'd be a Catholic kneeling there praying for my sick child.

One of my very favorite churches is the Jesuit Church located on Baronne Street. In the back right corner of the church is a memorial to Our Lady of Prompt Succor. She is particularly revered in New Orleans for turning the British back in the Battle of New Orleans and halting a fire about to consume the Ursuline Convent. Sometimes Jimmie's mother would accompany me and stand before that statue to pray. During those times, I'd find myself thinking, "Please hear Mrs. Peltier's prayers. You know her well, and she means much more to you than I. I'd very much like to know you better, but one cannot just jump into a friendship."

Then there was the Holy Name of Jesus Church on St. Charles Avenue — the church where both Jim and I had been baptized. Attending Mass there always made me feel even more sad. Finally, there was the Mater Dolorosa Church on Carrollton Avenue near Oak Street.

I'm sure my running from church to church must have looked ridiculous to those in Heaven. People around me weren't aware I was visiting all these churches, but I'd have done anything to help Jim.

I'd never prayed before to a saint to intercede for me. My prayers had always been to God alone. I continued praying to God, but there were so many hours to fill in each day that one day, I began asking the saints to pray for us.

I tried to evaluate what I was doing as I wondered why my prayers weren't being answered. Even to me, I seemed frantic with so many thoughts racing inside my head. Perhaps I wasn't praying with enough faith. I knew some people had favorite saints they'd been praying to for years. Since I'd just learned about this new way to pray, maybe my prayers would be ineffective.

The Bible phrase about the parents' sins being inflicted on their children haunted me, forcing me to search my life. At twenty-one years of age and having grown up in the dry town of DeRidder as a God-fearing Baptist, I'd never committed a mortal sin. There were, of course, venial sins and so many shortcomings. Perhaps my impatience and my making demands of God were a serious shortcoming, so I tried to settle down and let God have His way.

Slowly I was beginning to realize God's plan just might not be the same one I had in mind. That sounds very immature and naïve now, but I'd never had a reason before to do this soul-searching. My praying for help and guidance during my school years so I'd do my best as I tackled each new task with an open mind was different from what I was now asking God. I felt so helpless and so alone, but I knew He was all-powerful. Before I knew it, I'd slip into begging again.

For a little piece of tubing in a child's neck to work didn't seem to be such a big request to grant when there were so many people on earth. All I wanted was to be able to slip back into daily living with my child and husband. Was this too much to ask of the God I loved so much?

I took notice of the people rushing around me. They didn't even seem to believe in God, yet they seemed happy. Many of them weren't even following the Ten Commandments, but they appeared to be healthy and busy. In spite of my feeling desperate at times, no one could tell by being with me what my thoughts were. However, I'm sure if they reflected after a visit, they could imagine my beginning discouragement.

By now, Jimmie and I had to take a second look at our situation. I surely couldn't go to Florida and leave the proximity of Jim's doctor. We didn't even know when Jim would be able to leave the hospital. Jimmie and I realized we'd have to do something for ourselves.

Jimmie went to his Chief Dental Officer and to the base commander of Patrick Air Force Base to request a compassionate transfer. We both wanted Jimmie to be assigned to a base closer to New Orleans so we'd be near Dr. Garcia. Although these two men understood Jimmie's dilemma, they scoffed at the possibility of a transfer. They didn't know my husband.

After leaving Patrick Air Force Base, Jimmie sent his request to the Air Force Research and Development Command in Washington. It would then go to the Pentagon for final approval and, finally, back down to the base again. This could take a very long time, if the request was granted at all.

Edwin Willis was the Congressman from our Louisiana district. Since my husband knew him personally, Jimmie asked Congressman Willis for help. Congressman Willis was very cooperative and sent out memos to each stop along the way, asking if the order had been approved, and if not, why not, and if so, please get on with it without delay.

During the time this request for a compassionate transfer was being considered in Washington, Jimmie and I were particularly concerned because we couldn't foresee our future. The friends who'd invited me to live in their home while I was in New Orleans suddenly asked me to leave. What a shock that was! They'd sought me out and insisted I use a vacant room in their home. That room was isolated from the rest of the house and had its own private entrance. I was seldom there, using the room only to sleep, and I did pay rent. The discouragement of our having a sick child and the helplessness of our situation were touching more people's lives all the time.

My friends weren't angry with me. All of the commotion about Jim's illness had begun to depress their twenty-year-old daughter who lived at home. For that reason, they thought it best for me to find lodging elsewhere.

I certainly tried to understand their problem. This time in our life was hard for everyone, and more than anyone, I wished it would go away. Nevertheless, having this new burden added to the uncertainty of our situation wasn't easy.

However, I was amazed at the calmness with which I faced this new problem. I'm surprised even now I could be thrown from pillow to post and still welcome each new day with hope. I simply decided to move into Jim's hospital room. There didn't seem to be a need for a private duty nurse any longer. I'd learned to recognize a real problem with hydrocephalus as well as anybody, and I certainly loved feeding my baby and caring for him all by myself.

Thinking positively helped. I always tried to do things for myself instead of pushing the call button for the nurse. Because I was a dietician, I felt more at home than I'd have had I not been so familiar with hospitals.

One day, a "nurse" came into Jim's room. We had many visitors, so that was nothing unusual. People hearing of this baby who'd been in the hospital for weeks would come by to see us. This "nurse" offered to stay with Jim while I went out for his afternoon bottle. I thought it kind of her, got his bottle, thanked her, and thought nothing more of it. About three hours later when I wanted to buy a sandwich for supper, I found my wallet missing.

That caused a lot of excitement for a while, and the hospital was in a turmoil. When I went to the police station to identify that "nurse," I learned she'd been doing this in hospitals throughout New Orleans – Baptist Hospital, Touro Infirmary, Hotel Dieu Hospital and Ochsner Foundation Hospital. In each scenario, she entered the hospital room dressed as a nurse and offered to help. Being in need, sick people responded to her kindness. Then she stole their wallets. She admitted to the thefts and said she had quickly removed the money and discarded the wallets in wastebaskets. She also admitted having stolen from a room with a little boy who had a big head.

*****

Finally, Jimmie's transfer orders arrived. Biloxi it was to be. My mother came to stay with Jim in the hospital while I went by train to Coca Beach, Florida, for a short visit and to help pack all of our furnishings for the move. Jimmie and I drove back together to Keesler Air Force Base in Mississippi. Having a glimpse at the outside world again felt wonderful. The hospital had become a prison, more of a prison for my mind than for my body.

The friends my dental officer husband had made were refreshing. After socializing with adults in the outside world a few times, I began to think more like them. For a few days, I experienced an ordinary life as I made seafood gumbo for Jimmie's friends or shared a pot of coffee with them. As I packed for the move, we talked about trivial everyday things, and my courage returned. The hospital room was so narrow and circumscribed; it had shrunken the scope of my life. I'd forgotten how great it was to be around laughter. My hope was revived.

The trip back to New Orleans was wonderful because I was with Jimmie. My love for him had grown with all that was happening to us. The love I thought had been complete grew with our suffering. We never dwelt on our adversities when we were together; instead, we tried to have meaningful conversations, to laugh, and to have fun. We'd both been born happy people. In spite of all that was happening, we made a conscious effort not to be martyrs and remained happy.

Jimmie could hardly wait to see Jim. His face was unguarded for a few moments when he saw how much larger Jim's head had grown. Even with the periodic taps to relieve the pressure, fluid had still been collecting, and the bones had been pushed farther apart. Because I had been with Jim every day, I hadn't noticed how much his head had grown. Now, after being away for a few days, I saw with Jimmie's eyes.

I thanked God for the emotions I saw Jimmie feel when Jim began to smile and respond to his attention. Although Jimmie's heart broke at seeing Jim's head so much larger, his eyes lit up as he began to enjoy knowing his son. Even then, Jim had a strong personality and an active body. His eyes were alert, never downcast, as many hydrocephalics' eyes are. He learned to enjoy and, indeed, demand the attention he got from his over-eager audience.

When a sick child smiles, a parent feels a pride that is difficult to explain. Maybe it is less pride than joy at seeing one's child happy in spite of his condition. It is a special feeling Jimmie and I shared many times.

Because all three of us were together, the days that stretched endlessly before us seemed less miserable. And Jim was actually better. His tube was working without interruption.

Jimmie went on to Biloxi to check in at the airbase and to get settled temporarily in the Bachelor Officers' Quarters. I felt much better knowing he was only a hundred miles away instead of a thousand.

One day at the very end of September, Dr. Garcia announced that since Biloxi was only one hour away and we seemed to understand hydrocephalus and the symptoms associated with a shunt not working well, Jim could leave the hospital.

We thanked God for this blessing. Thanksgiving was a welcome respite from all the prayers of supplication we had offered. On October 2, 1954, one hundred days after Jim's admission to Mercy Hospital, we drove together to Biloxi.

Chapter Five

Keesler Air Force Base

*J*immie and I were assigned a vacant home at 406 Pinelawn Street. The little duplex was just off Keesler Air Force Base, and our furniture had arrived from Florida. Feeling part of the human race again, we launched into one of the happiest times of our lives.

Jim had outgrown his ribboned bassinette. What fun it was to buy a baby bed and a new set of pacifiers. Jim took everything in stride, and we were very happy.

For six long months, I'd been a party to emotions my young years had never had reason to demand before. I'd begged God for help. I'd felt despair when He didn't answer my prayers. Then I had begun to wonder about God's will, realizing His will and what I wanted might not be the same. That had been a very disturbing and unacceptable thought. How could He not want Jim to be well?

Now such questions faded from my mind. For the time being, God seemed to have answered my prayers. To finally leave Mercy Hospital as a family to share our first home felt great. Thanking Him profusely, I gave God all the credit. After having been isolated and feeling so discouraged, we were finally out in the world, lost among all the other average, normal people. Maybe we could stay that way. I felt certain our happiness wouldn't bother anyone, especially God.

As Jimmie and I warmed bottles of formula and used the baby presents that had been packed away for six months, we tried to integrate ourselves into Keesler Air Force Base's military society.

We found stretchable caps that could cover Jim's head to keep him warm. Since Jim couldn't hold his head up, we found a stroller that allowed him to lie back at an angle. He was alert and interested in everything surrounding him. The world was now visible to him from the sidewalk.

Our neighbors learned to love Jim as the special baby on the block. He had a way of giving everyone his total attention. Because he wasn't able to crawl and explore his surroundings physically, he did it through his eyes alone. He had a way of demanding to be noticed — not by crying, but by what looked like sincere interest in each person.

Except for his large head, Jim was gorgeous. Each day, his body was growing to catch up with his enlarged head. We frequently measured his head, calculating the average size of a normal man's head, how much a child's head usually grows in a life span, and figuring that if there were no more abnormal growths, then he'd appear normal when he became a man.

The days weren't long enough for our happiness. Jim slept well, and all three of us played together in our bed in the mornings. Jim and I looked forward to our Captain Peltier's return home for lunch and dinner. Jimmie was home by four o'clock every afternoon, and we all made the most of every minute.

To now pray with thankfulness rather than with desperate asking was a joy. Even though the three of us went to daily Mass as often as possible, our priest assured me that staying home doing my duties in God's name was as pleasing to God as attending church daily.

Finally, I could put my dietetic training into practice. Cooking and cleaning my kitchen offered me the normal life the hospital had stolen all these three months. Even doing everyday duties like cleaning bathrooms was marvelous after my having been deprived of them. I really felt I was living my dream of a little white house with a picket fence around it that locked out all life's unpleasantries.

*****

Jimmie has always made friends easily. He has a strong personality and a great gift for making people laugh. Through him, I met many lovely people.

Placed in a situation not of their choosing, people in the armed services seem more outgoing and open than they might be back home where friends had already been made, and they may not have a need to be as friendly. They have an extra drive to be nice to their fellow officers. Because of that, Jimmie's fellow dental officers saw our problem in the right light and treated us like any other family with a child. They invited Jimmie to play golf, and we met them often at the Officer's Club for brunch or happy hour. Our family fit in at Keesler. Being normal again was great!

One day, Jimmie asked me to go to the Officer's Club for a party. My first thought was, *I can't leave Jim!*

But I thought again. Our life together as husband and wife was already challenged by our children's illness. I knew if I chose always staying with our baby in lieu of going out with my husband, I'd regret it. Staying home with Jim was very tempting, but I made a very difficult decision that day. I'd find competent help to keep my baby, and I'd always go with Jimmie wherever he asked me to go. I wasn't going to force him to go out alone.

Jimmie was also having a very hard time, and I was wise enough to know a man so good-looking with so much to offer having a wife who felt she could never leave home because of a baby could easily find other interests. I vowed to myself I'd go with Jimmie every time he asked — no matter what! I knew he'd never want to go anywhere if the situation indicated we should stay home. After all, we were only a telephone call away from Jim. So we went to that party and enjoyed every minute of it.

On one of these calm, happy days, Jim suddenly vomited. It was projectile vomiting; one of the symptoms of hydrocephalus was back. Jimmie and I rushed Jim back to New Orleans for Dr. Garcia to tap his head. Again we entered Mercy Hospital, and again the interminable waiting began. Jim's shunt seemed to work for a time, but just as we'd become encouraged, he'd need another tap.

After Jim had been hospitalized for three weeks, Dr. Garcia walked in one morning, announcing he was being called into the United States Navy and would be stationed in Pensacola, Florida.

What a shock this was! How frightening! We considered Dr. Garcia a very necessary part of our lives. Our child couldn't survive without the removal of excess fluid when it accumulated. There was no way to predict when this might happen, and at that time, Keesler Air Force Base didn't have a neurosurgeon on staff. This seemed to be an impossible situation.

Because Jimmie was in the Air Force, we surmised we'd be allowed to use the Pensacola Naval Base Hospital. A few days later, Dr. Garcia reported for duty, and I prepared to follow him to Pensacola.

Our families had been faithful throughout our stay at Mercy Hospital, visiting us regularly and giving us their love and support. We all began to realize, however, that Jim's illness was ongoing. Our families had to stay home and hold their lives together, limiting their time with us to major crises. As Jim's parents, we felt each crisis was major, but obviously, some were more critical than others. We knew this move was one we'd have to handle without any help from our families. Jimmie felt he needed to save his three-day passes until critical situations arose because our future was very much in doubt. In order to save those passes for a rainier day, I went to Florida alone.

Fortunately, Jimmie's dental classmate and a very close friend, Wally Nicaud, and his wife, Emily, were stationed in Pensacola. Their home offered a place where I could bathe and relax and have someone to talk to, and it was good for Jimmie to know someone in Pensacola could help me when needed.

The pediatric ward at the Pensacola Naval Base Hospital was one very large room filled with baby beds. Parents weren't allowed to stay with their children. Dr. Garcia, in his very undefiable way, stated, "Mrs. Peltier will stay with her son. She will not bother you, and she, alone, knows when the baby has an emergency. When she tells you to call me, call me, wherever I am."

With that, I moved in. Having only a pillow available, I slept on the floor under Jim's bed at night. Occasionally during Jim's naps, I would slip over to my friend's home for a bath and a chance to phone Jimmie.

On one of those mid-afternoon visits to take a bath, I started experiencing terrific abdominal cramps. I believe I suffered a miscarriage, so I conditionally baptized what I believe was the fetus. I hadn't visited a doctor to confirm my pregnancy, but from all indications, I feel sure I had been pregnant. After resting a while, I felt better and hurried back to the hospital. There was no time to think very much about it.

During all this time, Jim acted like any other normal seven month old baby, laughing and playing with the mobile hanging over his bed. Just a slightly enlarged head and a little shaved spot on top of his head with merthiolate on it gave evidence of the last tap.

One day, Jim's eyes began to be slightly downcast, and before he could move on to the next symptom of projectile vomiting, I immediately asked the nurse to call the doctor. Dr. Garcia was true to his word.

Minutes later, Dr. Garcia walked into Jim's room in his casual, yet authoritative manner. He said, "Good morning, Mother," and then took Jim into a glass-enclosed room to relieve Jim's pressure. I sat and waited in my usual manner. This time I could have peeked, but running away from this situation was easier, so I chose not to look.

Following the procedure, Dr. Garcia walked away in his

slow, determined manner. Later, I found out by accident that he'd been in surgery, operating on a young naval pilot who had just crashed. He had actually left in the middle of surgery to take care of my son!

Dr. Garcia's family was still in New Orleans while he looked for adequate housing for them in Pensacola. On weekends, he went back home to New Orleans to be with them.

Since we had to have Dr. Garcia readily available, Jimmie would come to Pensacola, drive me and Jim back to New Orleans, and help check Jim into Mercy Hospital for the weekend.

By now, it looked as if the Torkildson procedure wasn't working because the frequency of the cerebral fluid build-up began to increase. Jimmie came in from Biloxi one weekend while I was in New Orleans with Jim. While we were both present, Dr. Garcia told us Jim needed further surgery. He explained his unexpected induction into the Navy made it impractical for him to be Jim's neurosurgeon and suggested we find another doctor.

Not many brain surgeons were interested in performing hydrocephalic procedures in New Orleans or anywhere else during 1954. Several names were mentioned in our discussions, but when we asked Dr. Garcia what decision he felt we should make, he replied, "If he were my child, I would go to the Children's Hospital in Boston. Dr. Donald Matson is there, and they're making big strides in this field. The hospital has a ward just for pediatric neurosurgery."

When we heard Dr. Garcia's advice, we knew we were headed for Boston. We had to have the best for Jim. The sooner we'd get Jim to Boston the better, so we immediately made reservations on a night flight. Thank goodness for that three-day pass! Jimmie could fly up with me over the weekend and then come back to the base.

It was December and cold where we were headed, so I dashed out to buy a few warm clothes. Before we left that evening for Boston, Jimmie gave me my Christmas present — a diamond bracelet. Christmas was still two weeks away, but

I think he wanted to cheer me up and knew how much the bracelet would mean to me. For a moment, I felt a little guilt at finding joy in a material object at a time like this, but since I'm a romantic, I appreciated such a gift from my husband because it meant he was thinking of me. Not knowing what we might encounter next, we cherished those few happy interludes.

As Jimmie and I prepared for our departure from Mercy Hospital that evening, Dr. Garcia removed the fluid from Jim's head. We gathered together all Jim's x-rays to take with us. Jimmie asked Dr. Garcia to give us names of a few places and a written order just in case Jim got into trouble and needed a tap before we reached Boston.

I was amazed at how matter-of-factly we accepted this new turn of events. Once again, there were no tears. Once again, we called to inform our parents of the situation and found them to be understanding. Once we were caught up in this whirlwind, we just did whatever the next day demanded of us. I really believe God gave us that strength because we never sat around feeling sorry for ourselves. We did what had to be done while sharing our strength and our love with our son.

Chapter Six

Boston Children's Hospital

Jimmie and I bundled Jim up in those great little-boy pajamas since we were traveling at night and hoped he might sleep. At five o'clock we left Mercy Hospital for Moisant International Airport. Jim did sleep for a long time on the plane as we relaxed.

Then he awakened, and there appeared the dreaded symptoms of increased pressure — downcast eyes, being cross, crying, and then Jim spit out his pacifier that always consoled him.

There were no jet airplanes in 1954, only big four-engine propeller airplanes. The flight was not today's two-hour long flight to New York; it was four and one-half hours long. The minutes seemed to drag by. We knew if the pressure wasn't treated, Jim could go into a coma or suffer brain damage and possibly die!

Jimmie asked the pilot to radio ahead for transportation as we quickly decided to get off in New York City. It was now two o'clock in the morning. We knew we had to get help for Jim as quickly as possible even though we very much wanted to go to Boston where we were expected.

New York was bitterly cold. Jimmie and I pulled our coats tightly around us and climbed into a taxi for a cold, lonely ride through the dark streets to find the New York Neurological

Institute. We wondered if there'd be a doctor on night duty who could tap Jim's head. We didn't know whether those in charge at the institute would call a doctor or whether they'd even help us at all.

I'm sure this was much harder for Jimmie than for me since he was the one looking after us. Jimmie is a very confident person. Because he's a doctor, I always felt he could take care of any situation, but now we were on unknown ground. We needed help soon and didn't have time for a lot of unnecessary explanations or red tape.

When Jim was under no pressure, he could make us feel good, even when situations were discouraging. But when he was under pressure, as he was now, we were frightened beyond endurance.

At last, we reached the big, tall monument of a building called the Neurological Institute and began the sobering experience of entering the emergency room. The doctor present carefully studied Jim's x-rays and the papers we had with us. Then he began a thorough, deliberate examination which seemed to last forever as he examined Jim's eyes with a light. Jim was getting more and more upset because of his discomfort.

Finally, Jimmie pleaded, "Someone has got to do something before he gets worse. Please help him!"

Following Jimmie's outburst, the doctor replied, "Well, I'm a neurologist and can't do the procedure, but I'll get someone who can."

Our hearts fell because this meant someone else would be doing a complete physical examination before he would tap Jim's head. The minutes were becoming critical.

This is when we learned the meaning of intelligent compassion. The second doctor recognized Jim's problem immediately. Without any fanfare, off he went with Jim.

Throughout all our experiences with Dr. Garcia, Jimmie and I had learned to respect the care with which intracranial fluid should be removed. Only a certain amount must be slowly aspirated at one time, and it must be done slowly as the patient lies quietly for a time to adjust to the change in pressure.

After just a matter of minutes in that strange hospital, we looked up and saw the unknown doctor returning with Jim. We were stunned! The doctor was holding Jim in his arms in an upright position, and Jim was laughing.

We couldn't believe how depressed Jim's soft spot was. There must have been at least a half-inch depth between the bones on top of Jim's head, but he couldn't have looked happier!

As the sun came up that morning and we drove away from that big hulk of a building, all three of us were happy and laughing. We had triumphed over yet another impossible time.

After that experience in New York, Jimmie and I welcomed the thought of Boston. To have Jim in the care of a doctor in a place where someone was always near to help him seemed to be our only answer.

On our flight to Boston, Jim sat on Jimmie's knees. Each time the plane hit an air pocket, Jim giggled, amusing all the people around us. I always remember that sound when we're on planes and the rides are a little bumpy. When we finally arrived in Boston, we were all in good spirits.

Dr. Matson was very nice to us. He was familiar with Jim's history, having already heard about us from Dr. Garcia. While giving the admitting orders, he casually noted there were no visiting hours.

Not even for me?

No. The doctors would be available by phone every evening at five-thirty. We could call every day for current reports, and when Jim was ready for release, they'd let us know.

This was a real shock to both Jimmie and me. We'd assumed I'd be staying with our baby. However, we had learned during these past months that a person has to do what he has to do. Now we were being forced to practice that philosophy again. So we once again gave Jim to a nurse who'd put him in a bed in the glass-enclosed pediatric neurosurgery ward.

Jimmie and I took a long look through those glass panes.

We saw about sixteen beds filled with sick children. Some had a permanent needle in their heads to drain the excess fluid as it accumulated. Seeing these children distressed me the most because I feared my child would need this treatment.

We watched the nurses put Jim in the second bed on the right. When it was time for us to walk away, we tried to give the nurse Jim's pacifier. She refused. This was such a small thing we felt she could have done since that pacifier had given Jim such comfort in the preceding months when he had to lie in his bed all alone. Even if she had taken the pacifier to assuage our worry, the deception would have eased our pain. Jimmie and I tried not to be doting parents, but who would not try to squeeze in every helpful trifle at this point?

As Jimmie and I walked through the snow under Jim's window four stories above, we could hear him screaming. There were no other city noises around us to block or dull that sound. That piercing, troubled cry we had learned to know too well resounded in our ears. Before, we could always run to Jim to try to help him, but now we were locked out of his life.

Jimmie and I were stuck in one of those situations where we had no control, one of those times when all we could do was try to summon the courage to keep walking. As we silently walked away, Jimmie and I held each other's hand.

*****

Dr. Matson had made reservations for us at the Peter Brent Brigham Hotel because it was close to the hospital. The hotel was a very unique place. Pointing out to one another its unusual features helped to distract Jimmie and me. The elevator had a wrought iron cage we could look out as we ascended. It must have been one of the first elevators made. At the end of each hall, big buckets of water stood ready to be used in case of a fire. As we sat in the dining room with its high vaulted ceilings, we ordered the boiled New England dinner, not a very appetizing meal to us South Louisianans.

That night Jimmie and I slept in our old-fashioned hotel

room in the same city block as Jim. We waited the next day to make the 5:30 p.m. call, but after that, there was nothing else we could do. Since we weren't allowed to visit Jim, we knew we should go home.

Because we had two more days before Jimmie had to report to Keesler, we spent them in New York City. We held hands as we walked the snow-covered streets, trying to make the best of a very bad situation.

Christmas was near, and seeing the Christmas tree at Rockefeller Center in all its beauty filled us with a confusion of many sad and happy thoughts. We didn't do a lot of talking. Instead, we tried to be aware of the beauty around us. One thing was certain — we knew Christmas was going to bring a new meaning and a new dimension in this, our first year with our own child.

Before, we always spent Christmas in Thibodaux at the Peltier family home, a colonial-type mansion facing Bayou Lafourche. It's the kind of home one likes to think of when picturing the grand style of living in the South. Tall, stately columns support the roof over the veranda, the very necessary porch that shades the thick walls and makes the home cooler. A large wide door looks inviting to passers-by.

Having all of the Peltier family gather there for the holidays was customary. Because I was an only child, I felt these occasions were more exciting for me than anyone else. This Christmas, the senior Peltiers had eleven grandchildren. With all the family present, twenty-two of us gathered after Mass for Christmas dinner at the long dining table. Afterwards, everyone exchanged presents.

Because we'd been living away, Jimmie and I felt secure being welcomed into a large family Christmas. We joined in all the laughter and fun of the day, ate the big turkey dinner with dirty rice and all the trimmings, and were as joyful as we could possibly be without our son. Everyone was aware that Jim was far away in the Boston hospital, so there was no need to discuss this. Each relative wanted everyone present

to celebrate the real meaning of Christmas with the love God
wanted us to share.

Chapter Seven

Waiting

$\mathcal{E}$ach day at 4:30 p.m. our time, Jimmie and I called the Boston hospital for news regarding Jim. The preoperative tests were having normal results, and Jim's surgery was scheduled. Then one day, the doctor reported Jim and all the other pediatric patients in the ward had come down with chicken pox. They seemed to think Jim might have been the carrier. We weren't sure of his having been exposed to chicken pox, but there might have been a case of chicken pox in the Pensacola hospital. However, there was certainly nothing we could do about it. Because of this unfortunate turn of events, Jim's hospital stay was prolonged.

On January 16, the doctors tried to drain Jim's excess fluid by using a ventriculo-cervical shunt, a device similar to a Torkildson shunt. When that didn't drain, the doctors decided to remove one of Jim's kidneys and connect the shunt tubing to his ureter, the tube going from his kidney to his bladder. The fluid would then drain through his urine directly out of his body. The length of tubing would offer some post drainage while the ureter would actually offer suction to assist the drainage.

At the time, Boston Children's Hospital had been having success with this type of surgery. Although this procedure sounded very complicated to Jimmie and me, we were totally committed to the doctors' judgment and agreed to whatever the experts there suggested.

Jimmie and I continued our daily 4:30 p.m. calls for news about our son. Because only one hour was allowed for all the children's families to call for information, our conversations were short. We were probably the first ones to call each afternoon because our days were built around those calls, and I allowed nothing to distract me.

Secretly, I wondered how on earth a mother could love two babies. I loved Jim so much that I wondered if there could be enough love to go around for a second child. I also wondered if other mothers felt this way. Though I was ashamed to ask, I'd soon find out.

Late that December, Jimmie and I suspected I was pregnant again. When it was confirmed, we were both thrilled. We'd been assured having two children with hydrocephalus was virtually impossible, so we felt confident we wouldn't have another child with this terrible condition.

Back at Keesler Air Force Base, Jimmie and I used this time to get to know people better. We were invited to many barbecues and took our turn at the backyard grill as well. We became very well acquainted with Father Enright and Father Graft, Keesler's two Catholic chaplains, and spent many pleasant hours with them.

Because over twenty thousand of their parishioners were eighteen-year-olds who'd just entered the armed services and had never before been away from home, being chaplains at the Air Force base wasn't easy for Father Enright and Father Graff. These airmen's problems were unbelievable and often unsolvable, so the two priests found some respite from those unusual problems by visiting with us.

Being in the presence of those two chaplains God had chosen to do His work on earth was a comfort. They, of course, had no answers to give us, but having them share their time with us helped our mental outlook immeasurably. Because I needed and wanted my prayers answered so badly, I was in awe of anyone who dedicated his life to Christ. I always believed priests must have a more direct line to God than I had and felt Father Enright and Father Graff would be able to influence God to cure Jim.

Finally, we received the call from Boston saying Jim could come home. Oh, happy day! Jim was so glad to see us as we dressed him in the clothes we'd brought. As the nurses handed him to us, our future seemed simple. Although our son had been away from us for almost six weeks, he acted as though we'd never been out of his sight when he was back in our arms.

Considering the importance of the instructions for Jim's postoperative care, our conversation with the doctors was unusually brief. They told us because of the delay caused by his having chicken pox, Jim had been connected to a needle that provided continuous drainage of the excess fluid from his head during the weeks before he was able to have surgery performed. After the ventriculo-ureteral (head to ureter) shunt was in place, Jim experienced convulsions because of salt loss in his body, but a proper daily diet had corrected this problem. Some of these details had not been voiced during our daily telephone conversations with the doctors, so Jimmie and I were hearing them for the first time.

Because the intracranial fluid would be excreted from his body through urination, Jim would now be losing every day two essentials — sodium and chlorine. These two important electrolytes would have to be replaced daily with table salt. We were to add to his food each day one teaspoonful of salt divided into small amounts. I'd need to carefully measure the salt each morning to make sure he had the proper intake. Then, the doctors casually added, we'd need to bring Jim back after his growing ten or so inches to have his tube replaced. To Jimmie and me, this wasn't a minor point!

As the three of us flew back to Louisiana, Jim's smiles and laughs brought us much joy. Other than having a shaved head, he wasn't even weak after his stay at the Boston hospital. Once we settled in the plane, we gave Jim his pacifier. He sucked on it a few times, took it out, looked at it, and quickly popped it back into his mouth. To be perfectly honest, he was much less spoiled than when we had left him. Within only a few days, however, he was back in the swing of making us jump around to please him.

Adding salt to Jim's diet was not much of a problem. Putting a tiny bit in his milk, meat, and vegetables was easy, but hominy grits was the food where I could always hide the most salt. So like a true southerner, Jim ate his grits every day.

Because 1955 was a really bad year for mosquitoes in Biloxi, I had to carefully choose the time of day for Jim's daily strolls in the sun. During our daily excursions, all the children on the block began to know Jim well again, and he was always thrilled to be around people. Another of Jim's favorite pastimes was riding in the car. Because I was pregnant, very nauseated, and wanted to keep busy, the two of us spent many happy hours riding up and down the beach in Biloxi.

Jimmie and I had a special high chair built for Jim that was placed in the middle of a folding table that was similar to a card table and rolled around. The back of the chair was taller than usual and had slanted sides to help support Jim's head. Everything was well padded with leather.

Jim could sit in the chair and play with his toys on the table or try to feed himself. When sitting in his special high chair or his stroller with its slanted headpiece to hold his head, Jim could be in the center of everything. And that was where he wanted to be.

*****

Jimmie was one of fifty-five dentists on Keesler Air Force Base practicing dentistry. He enjoyed being a dentist, but his hard work often went unappreciated, making it less rewarding than it should have been. Many doctors and officers asked Jimmie to take care of their dental needs because he was doing such outstanding work, but most of his work was on young men very new to military service.

After completing one extremely difficult full-mouth rehabilitation in which he took particular pride, Jimmie questioned his life's plan of practicing general dentistry.

After discharging his prized patient at closing time, Jimmie changed from his white dental coat to his captain's uniform and walked out on the porch to wait for his carpool ride. He looked completely different in uniform wearing his cap. Sitting there on the bench was his prized patient saying to a buddy, "That SOB dentist just messed me up!" I wish I had been there to hear Jimmie dress that corporal down.

With this experience fresh in his thoughts, Jimmie began to consider becoming an oral surgeon. Fortunately, the one qualified and two partially trained oral surgeons on the base allowed him to observe their work and talked with him about the additional years required to specialize in this area. The more Jimmie observed them and the more he thought about it, the more he knew this is what he wanted to do. Once he was sure, he began planning the program that would take him in this new direction.

While Jimmie was discovering he wanted to become an oral surgeon, our lives were settling into a comfortable routine. We had to give Jim his daily addition of sodium and chloride. If he experienced any vomiting or had other interference getting and retaining these ions, he would go into electrolyte imbalance very quickly. That spelled trouble.

Jimmie and I noticed when Jim cried unusually hard, his gag reflex activated and caused him to vomit easily. This active gag reflex was probably the result of his frequent vomiting episodes. Some nights when he cried and cried, we were unable to quiet him. On those occasions, out we would go, pajamas and all, for a ride in the car to try to make him happy. We were willing to do anything to prevent Jim from throwing up, regardless of the cost. In the middle of a two o'clock in the morning ride once, Jimmie and I laughed at ourselves that a child dominated us so completely that we would be joy riding at such an ungodly hour.

Because of Jim's hyperactive gag reflex, we naturally tried to prevent his exposure to any disease. Even having a cold and being congested caused him to gag. Fever could cause brain swelling and could also result in his discomfort and vomiting.

Just when Jimmie and I thought we had all fairly well stabilized, Jim suffered a series of severe vomiting spells in the spring of 1955. We dashed over to the base hospital to see the pediatrician there. In just a matter of hours, Jim was so dehydrated that when we picked up his skin between our fingers, there was no elasticity.

Infusions of replacement fluids began immediately. However, Jim became unconscious even while receiving the replacement fluids. Hour after hour, he remained unresponsive. In those days, there were no sophisticated machines to measure the loss and replacement of electrolytes in that complicated system called electrolyte imbalance. The pediatrician needed to make mental calculations from a limited test available at that time. I remember that pediatrician was Jewish, was from the east, and was very capable and kind.

I had never seen Jimmie so totally discouraged as when we sat outside on the back steps of the hospital and prayed. Because I hadn't been around patients as much as Jimmie had, I didn't realize how near to death Jim was. Jimmie promised then that if God would let Jim live, he would attend Mass every day for the rest of his tenure in the service. This was no easy promise. The chapel wasn't close to our house. Jimmie would have to fast after midnight in order to receive Communion and get up before six every day.

Although the pediatrician tried several chemical combinations, Jim still didn't respond. Hours stretched on. Suddenly, Jim was better. A mother can tell the minute her child feels better. I knew Jim was going to be all right. After about twenty-four hours, his eyes began to sparkle again, and he began to smile. Jimmie and I knew our son was well once again.

Jimmie remained true to his promise of attending Mass daily even though it was difficult for us. All our plans had to be made or altered around Jimmie's Mass schedule. Because he was seen so often at church, everyone assumed he was a pillar of the church and asked him to serve on special committees. One committee had taken on the task of collecting money for a much-needed new church in the back bay area of Biloxi. Jimmie accepted this challenge with enthusiasm and did his part to make this new church a reality.

*****

Every chance Jimmie and I had, we visited our parents. While we were in DeRidder with my family that Easter, Jim vomited. We hurried to the local hospital. We knew the doctor there, and he recognized Jim's problem immediately. He gave Jim fluid through a needle placed into his muscle instead of his vein.

Because we had gotten to the hospital quickly enough, Jim's need for fluids was quickly supplied, and this crisis was over within thirty minutes. As usual, as soon as Jim felt better, he showed it with his big smiles. We were relieved, but there was no denying we had dodged lightning.

Time passed quickly. Before we knew it, Jim had grown four inches in height. It was time to take him back to Boston to have the shunt extension before it would pull out and stop working. This surgery wasn't as complicated as the surgery to insert the original shunt because the doctors didn't have to bother the ends of the tubing securely attached in the previous surgery. During this second operation, an extra length of tubing would be spliced into the first tube even though Jim felt well.

Following a long flight to Boston on July 11, Jim was admitted to the hospital. Jimmie and I returned to Biloxi and resumed the daily telephone calls for news regarding our son's condition. The surgery to lengthen the tubing was performed on July 25. All seemed well.

However, Jimmie and I were surprised when the doctors informed us on August 3 that they decided to remove the old ventricular-cervical shunt from Jim's neck because it was no longer needed. So Jimmie and I sat by the telephone on the day of Jim's surgery because the doctor would be the one to initiate the call after this surgery's completion.

On August 9, Jim was discharged, and Jimmie and I were there to take him home. I never could become accustomed to the idea of dropping our baby off and picking him up a month later after his having such traumatic surgery.

✝

Chapter Eight

Benita Ann

*O*nly eight days after our return from Boston with Jim, my labor pains began. Jimmie called his cousin Dottie Toups, a nurse in Thibodaux. Dottie drove alone to Biloxi to help us. Having Dottie around was wonderful because nurses have that special knack of making a mother more comfortable.

After being admitted to the hospital in Biloxi, I was placed in a ward where one woman had her baby in her bed before she could be taken into the delivery room. Another woman was screaming because she was afraid she, too, might deliver in her bed. Because of all of this excitement, my labor pains suddenly stopped.

Instead of discharging me, my obstetrician chose to intravenously induce labor. On August 17, 1955, Jimmie and I had our little girl. I named her Benita Ann, after me. She seemed to be in perfect health. Actually, she was an unusually beautiful baby. People from all over the hospital asked to see her because she was so pretty. Her hair was blonde; her skin was very fair; and her features were perfect. Of course, we checked her fontanel immediately. It proved to be normal, and Jimmie and I were ecstatic. Jim had just had his shunt revision and was doing well. Now he had a little sister.

Three glorious, busy weeks passed before Benita Ann's fontanel began to show a slight change. We called Dr. Al Hurst,

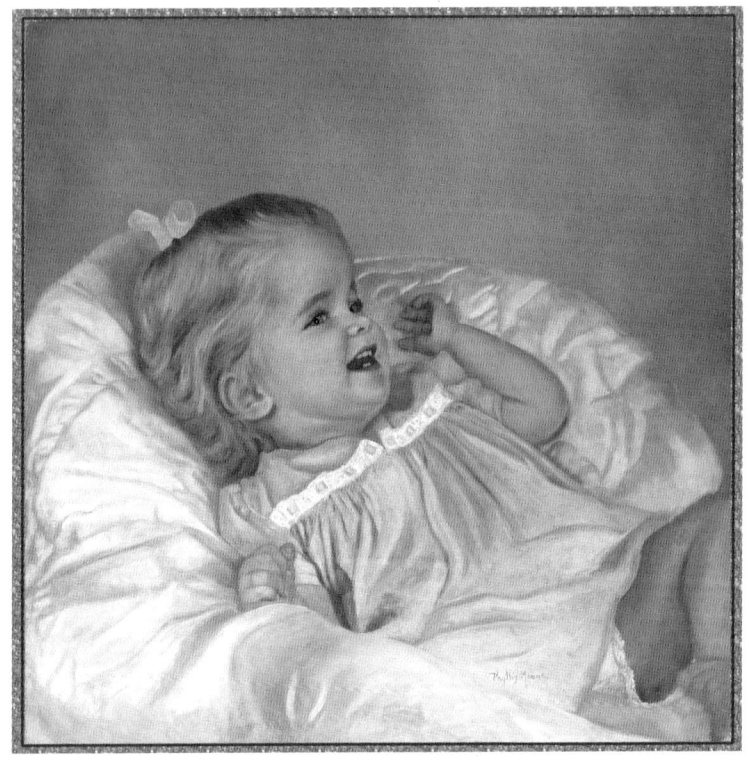

Benita Ann Peltier

a neighbor in the service. He said, "No, it's not so."

But a few days later, our worst fears were realized — our beautiful baby, Benita Ann, had hydrocephalus.

This nearly undid me. Jimmie and I couldn't comprehend how our beautiful little girl could have hydrocephalus. We dreaded that she'd have to face the surgeries and suffering having this terrible condition requires. Most of all, our hearts broke for Benita Ann as we thought of what this would mean to her — physically and emotionally. There'd be no normal home life for her. Instead, her life would be made up of hospitals and people in white uniforms. We wished we could have had the sickness instead of her. Everything seemed so useless and unnecessary, but we refused to give up hope entirely.

Then we thought of ourselves and what this would mean to our life. Jim required all of our thoughts and energies for one and one-half years. We wondered how we'd physically take care of two children with hydrocephalus. We'd have to once again begin the same uncertain path we'd traveled for so long.

Jimmie and I would again have to face the doctors with their guarded words and feelings. We would again have to wait outside closed doors within earshot of our baby crying while uncomfortable tests were being performed. We would again experience all the hospital admissions with long, seemingly unnecessary interviews in the hospital office and all the forms that would have to be filled.

Again my beautiful baby would be placed in a cold bed, and again I would be asked to step back while technicians came from all directions to do blood tests, urinalysis, and measure her precious head.

But most of all, we dreaded waiting outside swinging surgery doors for the eight and nine hour brain operations and those interminable days following the surgical procedure to see if the shunt would function. We'd be forced to helplessly watch another head grow and make a beautiful face change daily. With Jim, each step had been into the unknown. With

Benita Ann, Jimmie and I now knew all too well what each new step would bring. This felt even worse.

We had to face telling our parents the bad news one more time. At least Jimmie and I could get caught up in the day-to-day care of our babies, but our parents had to stay home and think about the tragedy of it all and wonder what was happening.

We worried about the bills – the doctor bills, the nursing bills, and the hospital bills that would follow. What money Jimmie and I had, we had hoped to spend on an office and a home for our little family. We were thankful, however, to be able to give our children the best of care.

We tried to fight the questioning and doubt in our minds, but these were ever present. One day I'd think, *All of those prayers, all of those times at church, all of those promises to God, yet this terrible pain again. Why?*

Then I'd sit on the sofa and think, *I've done nothing all of these years but love God. I'm not one of His friends who searches Him out only in trouble. I've been His friend all of my life — not a fair-weather friend. I've never had an identity crisis. I know my life is to be spent with Him after death. How can He allow this to happen to us?*

Then I'd busy myself for a few hours, only to begin wondering again, *Others who don't seem to know Him at all and others who don't seem to follow the commandments are in houses all over the world with healthy children.*

Again priests came, nuns came, all of the religious came to see us. Calls came from everywhere. People were praying for us. In my despair, I even questioned the effectiveness of prayers. So far, I hadn't found the answers I'd sought. Because I'd prayed all my life, I prayed again, not knowing what else to do. I began to pray for courage for Jimmie and me. I realized there'd be no miracle, and I knew there was no running from our situation. We had to face stark reality. No amount of asking questions, no amount of good wishes from others would help. Jimmie and I would have to stand alone and live through hydrocephalus one more time. Demands would be made of us I hoped we could meet. I prayed for strength.

Yet, there had been miracles. I'd read about so many in all the religious books. I remembered about the holy water others had administered. They received miraculous cures. I even tried pouring holy water over Benita Ann when the two of us were alone. I made all sorts of promises to God about all I'd do if only she could be cured.

I remembered reading that some parents had entered Holy Orders at the age of forty-five, separating to live their lives in the service of God. I even asked Jimmie if he thought doing this would help, but he knew nothing would help. We'd have to live though our situation just as it was. There was no escape.

We heard many pretty speeches. "How God must love you to send you these troubles." Others said, "He never sends you more than you can take." However, when we looked around at mental institutions, they all seemed to be filled with people who'd been sent more than they could take. Jimmie developed a real hatred for that platitude.

I guess I was born with the gift of faith, and for that, I'm thankful. From my early childhood, I loved the Lord. It was that simple. All these questions as to whether He sent the troubles or allowed the troubles to happen finally didn't matter. He certainly wasn't going to talk to me to give me any answers. I'd have to wait until my life ended for the answers to my questions, wanting God to explain a lot to me.

Out of all of my anguish came the realization I had problems and had to do my best to keep Benita Ann, Jim, and Jimmie as happy as I possibly could. And that, simply, was how I analyzed what I should do.

For three weeks prior to her diagnosis, Benita Ann was well. Three precious weeks. I truly enjoyed every minute. I nursed her and fed Jim and thought my world was complete. When I was holding Benita Ann and making faces to entertain Jim as he sat beside me in his special high chair, I wished the clock would stop. They loved me, and I loved them. I saw how wondrously easy it is for mothers to love more than one child.

Benita Ann was the prettiest baby we had ever seen. To sit and watch her head enlarge was very difficult. Her body was so small. Parents forget how tiny a newborn baby can be.

I don't know if having three happy weeks made the heartaches worse when we found out Benita Ann had hydrocephalus. We had to face making the telephone call to Boston to ask them to accept her as a patient. They preferred she be a little older before undergoing such a major procedure.

Both the days and our minds seemed hazy, yet the day seemed to pass all too quickly when we dressed Benita Ann in her pretty clothes for her trip to Boston. We'd traveled this road before and knew it well. This time our baby was even younger. She didn't even know us yet, which was a kind of blessing. At least she wouldn't miss us.

Benita Ann's admission to the hospital on September 18, 1955, seemed so routine to the doctors. I knew they had to protect themselves from being emotionally involved. Though I knew the doctors couldn't personally feel for each child they treated, at least not for long, I found it strange they could be so dispassionate. They asked many questions about our background for hints of genetic problems, but nowhere on either side had any of our relatives ever had a remotely similar problem.

We handed Benita Ann to the nurses. As she was placed into her bed in the glass-enclosed neurosurgical ward, Jimmie and I walked away once more. Benita Ann was one month old. Even though we'd already been on this road, it was no easier this second time.

Because there were two days left of Jimmie's three-day pass from Keesler, we came back through New York City to try to divert our thoughts. As Jimmie and I were walking along a New York street that night, we ran into a friend, Louis Roussel. A financial entrepreneur from New Orleans, Louis Roussel was an unusual person with an unforgettable character and had been born and reared just outside of Thibodaux.

Mr. Roussel told us he was entertaining all the Supreme Court judges from Louisiana for the Archie Moore – Rocky Marciano heavyweight championship fight in Yankee Stadium. The fight was a complete sellout, and rain had prevented it from taking place the night before in Yankee Stadium. Because he had two extra ringside tickets for the big fight, he insisted we join the party. We could pick up our tickets from another Louisianan, Abe Shushan.

Being in Mr. Shushan's elegant apartment in the Waldorf Astoria certainly gave us a chance to forget what was happening in Boston for a few minutes. So did being fortunate enough to meet all the Louisiana Supreme Court judges and attending the Archie Moore-Rocky Marciano fight.

Although it was over so quickly, the fight was something to share with the enormous crowd. I remember well one of Mr. Roussel's guests, a Louisiana Supreme Court judge sitting near us, as he said, "Jesus Christ! I haven't seen so many people since Huey Long's funeral!" That was Rocky Marciano's last heavyweight fight.

After that exciting New York interlude, Jimmie and I returned to Mississippi and built our life around the news from Massachusetts.

Jim, now one and a half years old, still needed a lot of extra attention. Unlike children his age, he had to spend most of his time sitting instead of walking around. So I had to entertain him during most of his waking hours. People were very nice to us, but our problems with sick children were beginning to be tiring for them. Friends and family who called often or wrote notes became discouraged. There was little left for them to say to offer comfort. I could understand why we had few visitors or contacts after people found out we had a second child with the same discouraging condition. Understanding, however, doesn't make things easier to accept.

*****

On September 21, 1955, Dr. Matson tried the ventriculo-cervical shunt on Benita Ann. That didn't work satisfactorily. So on October 14, he turned to a ventriculo-ureteral shunt just like Jim had. One of Benita Ann's kidneys was removed, and a plastic tube was connected to her ureter. This didn't work properly either, so the doctors had to revise it seven days later because the end connected to the ureter had come out of place. After that was corrected, the shunt adequately drained her head. After six weeks, we finally received the long-awaited call that Benita Ann could come home.

Benita Ann came home with the same orders as Jim — one teaspoonful of salt was to be given to her in her food daily. She was so young that she was still on formula. The milk from her bottle must have tasted terrible with salt added to it, but she drank it in spite of the taste.

Caring for two children with so little hope for a future would seem depressing, but Jimmie and I never really gave up. We always thought their surgeries would be successful and that they would, in time, lead normal lives. Jim and Benita Ann were so lovable. Maybe they needed more love than other babies so they'd feel secure when they had to face their pain. In our prayers, we turned everything totally over to God and His will as we continued playing our roles for Him. Jimmie still attended daily Mass, and we bathed, dressed and fed our two with as much love as any children ever had.

Television provided many happy hours for Jim. Captain Kangaroo and Mr. Greenjeans, along with Romper Room and the Mousketeers, amused him. Watching television was not Jim's only daily activity. He came with me to the grocery store, and, like all other little boys, he liked sitting in the grocery cart while I shopped. I never felt apologetic about his head size. He was so handsome and dear to me that I proudly took him everywhere.

Jimmie's family often came to spend time in Biloxi's resort area. They were so good to us. They took us out to eat and invited us to their hotel rooms so we could swim in the hotel pool. Although our thoughts were never put into words, we liked knowing they cared for us deeply enough to take this time to be with us. We always knew they supported us in our troubles through their caring and also knew they felt helpless because there was so little anyone could do.

Sometimes we took Jim and Benita Ann to visit our families just as if everything was normal. Cars weren't equipped with seatbelts in 1955. However, a wonderful contraption for the back of the car made traveling with babies easier. It hooked onto the back seat and formed a bed by connecting onto the front seat. This put our babies at window level so I could easily change their diapers and give them a bottle by kneeling on the front seat.

DeRidder was a little too far away from neurosurgeons, so Jimmie, the children and I went to Thibodaux more often because it was closer to the doctors we might need in case of an emergency. Coming home to a large family who loved us made us feel as if we belonged. I always felt the four of us were so alone, so those brief times of being included in a caring group was a particular solace to me. For some reason, I didn't feel as vulnerable when I was with our family.

Chapter Nine

Boston Again

$\mathcal{B}$y the beginning of 1956, I suspected I was pregnant again. Facing the nausea in an ordinary day is bad enough, but having two babies needing total care and constant attention made dealing with the morning sickness that sometimes lasted all day even harder.

However, Jimmie and I were happy again. Jim's and Benita Ann's shunts were both working well, and having my schedule running smoothly again was nice. We began to feel like a normal family once more.

But when I took Benita Ann out to sun on the steps after her bath that February day, I noticed she suddenly was no longer alert. When she didn't follow me with her eyes and lost all facial expression, I called Jimmie at work to tell him what had happened. He had learned to dread the page to answer the phone because there was scarcely any good news. Even though it was painful to call him again to give him this bad news, the only way we could go through this was by being honest with each other. Our always being truthful with each other helped us be strong in the knowledge that at least one other person carcd. By telling Jimmie, I was not relieving myself of the burden; instead, I was sharing it.

Jimmie and I had little choice but to return to Boston. We telephoned the doctors, trying to describe Benita Ann's symptoms, but the doctors couldn't help Benita Ann without seeing her.

Once again, we followed the same procedure — admitted our baby into Children's Hospital, returned to Biloxi, and again began our daily calls regarding her progress. Again, the doctor observed her for a few days and anticipated no need for surgery. About a week later, we were once again told the words we always dreaded hearing — Benita Ann was worse — she had meningitis.

Our baby was treated with massive doses of antibiotics for a week; after which, the doctors said she was well. When the hospital called notifying us Benita Ann could be discharged, Jimmie went to Boston alone to get her. I was so nauseated from this pregnancy that I stayed overnight with an aunt in New Orleans.

When time for the plane to arrive began to approach, I had to do a lot of fast talking to be allowed to take Jim with me to the airport. Our relatives thought they should either come with me or leave Jim with them while I went alone. I refused. For the four of us to be alone together was very important to me, so just the two of us met Jimmie and Benita Ann.

Even from a distance, I could tell something was wrong when I saw Jimmie walking toward us with Benita Ann in his arms.

He kept saying, "She can't see! The doctors gave her to me and didn't say anything about her condition. On the plane, I noticed she had a blank stare. I kept striking matches in front of her eyes and got no response. When I realized she couldn't see, I didn't know whether to get off the plane and go back to the hospital or just come on home. Then I thought, *To hell with those damn Yankees!* and came home."

The trip back home to Biloxi seemed to take forever. I let Jimmie talk out his feelings as I tried to grasp what this new development would mean. I was sorry he'd gone alone to Boston and had to face the realization of Benita Ann's blindness with no one present to share his shock and disappointment.

Our daughter was to be in total darkness for the rest of her life. We could do nothing but care for her. Although Benita Ann was unable to see, she still had a relaxed look on her face. She had such an angelic countenance as she lay in her bed rocking back and forth, smiling and making sounds that resembled a melody.

When we took Benita Ann to an opthalmologist to have her eyes examined, we learned there was nothing wrong with her eyes. Meningitis had damaged that part of her brain that enabled sight, and absolutely nothing could be done. Although we were never told, her being severely mentally handicapped was also obvious. Somehow we resumed the daily routine of our lives while trying to come to terms with Benita Ann's newest problem.

Gradually, Jimmie's idea of studying oral surgery had become more than just talk. He decided he definitely wanted to spend the additional three years required for this specialty. If he were accepted at Massachusetts General Hospital's oral surgery residency, he could train there so we would be in closer proximity to the neurosurgeon we needed to treat our children. He also investigated other noted oral surgery training programs located in areas known for their neurosurgical departments.

One was Duke University. A partially trained oral surgeon at Keesler had trained at Duke for one year and highly recommended their program. We then discovered Drs. Barnes Wodall and Guy Odom at Duke had actually taught Boston's Dr. Matson and were nationally recognized in the neurosurgical field. Knowing this, Jimmie applied to enter the Duke University Oral Surgery Residency program.

Having to accept we would be in another city away from family and friends for three years while Jimmie spent long hours in training was difficult. We had purchased a home in Thibodaux, and I had fully expected to return there after Jimmie completed his Air Force commitment. All this time, he had talked about going back to practice dentistry in his hometown. Going back home would also mean having our families near to help us with our sick children. Pregnant again, I just didn't see how I'd be able to face any more challenges or cope with any more changes over which we had no control.

With all his charm, Jimmie explained all his reasons for taking this step. When I realized how much this really meant to him and to our future together, I was able to agree although I'd have much preferred what I saw as the easier way.

When I'd signed the papers in DeRidder the Catholic Church required before I could marry Jimmie, I loved him so much I think I'd have agreed to anything to marry him as long as I obeyed God's commandments. Jimmie had literally swept me off my feet. His solid-type physique revealed his strength. His light green eyes glistened and danced with mischief, only to be outshined by his black, well-groomed hair and tan complexion.

Of course, his depth of character was the most exciting thing about him. A deep-thinking, compassionate person, Jimmie has always had an ardent love of God, which he integrated into his exciting life. His Acadian French origin made him into a romantic who loves to have fun, but who also works with a determination to get the most out of each hour. Just to be caught up in the momentum and intensity of Jimmie's way of living was thrilling. After my quiet, unassuming years of growing up, Jimmie represented all a vibrant man could bring to a loving wife. Being with him made me happy, and his presence in a room gave me a feeling of completeness.

Jimmie and I had given ourselves completely to each other every chance we had, but with the constancy of hydrocephalus, those times were few. We knew we needed a little time away. Jim and Benita Ann were holding their own and only needed love and care. My mother could give them that for a few days. The Air Force offered to give Jimmie leave to attend the American Dental Association meeting in San Francisco, California. Here was our chance to escape our routine though we loved our life with our family. We needed time for different thoughts and experiences. Jimmie and I loved each other and wanted to share romantic San Francisco together.

We knew God wanted us to be happy whenever we could. Although He had said to take up your cross, He didn't say anything about having to be sad. We felt our having fun together was pleasing to Him.

Daily we called home to check on our children and attended Mass. After that, we had fun. We loved holding on to the straps of the cable cars and climbing the steep hills of San Francisco. Dining in some of the famous gourmet restaurants at night was a treat. Laughing and talking about the trivial gave us a new way of thinking.

Refreshed and rejuvenated, Jimmie and I returned to Biloxi. After this trip, getting away for brief periods of time enabled us to handle our feelings of helplessness and the demands of raising children who weren't well. We needed a segment of life for ourselves to gain the balance to continue our struggles.

*****

Jimmie's military duty in the Air Force would terminate with his discharge in June. We waited to see if he'd be accepted into an oral surgery program. Our new baby was due in September, and I wouldn't allow myself to think about our future with another baby. With two hydrocephalics, surely we could never have another. If Jimmie was concerned about the health of our next baby, he didn't share his fears with me. Our days were too full caring for Jim and Benita Ann as we renewed our faith in God and waited. Time seemed to just move on.

Because Chaplain Graft had a special friend in Rome who was close to the Pope, he suggested we write a letter to Pope Pius XII asking him to pray for our baby we were expecting and telling him about the two children we already had. Chaplain Graft assured us the letter would reach the Pope's hands.

Much to our surprise, the Pope sent us his special blessing, saying he would remember us in his prayers and complimented us on our faith. We were touched by his beautiful letter.

Massachusettes General Hospital in Boston invited Jimmie to come up for an interview. Of course, we preferred a residency there because that's where our children had been treated and the doctors were familiar with our history. While waiting for word from Boston, Jimmie received a letter of acceptance from Duke University. He didn't want to reply too quickly because he first wanted to be sure about Boston.

When word did arrive from Boston, it was "no." Jimmie quickly accepted the residency at Duke, and we were making yet another turn in the long, winding road of our lives.

Chapter Ten

Durham, North Carolina

$\mathcal{A}$fter visits with our families in July, we packed, and with the aid of a quilted pad stretched across the back seat of the car, Jimmie and I drove with our babies to Durham, North Carolina.

Mattie Barnes, who'd worked so faithfully for us for two years in Biloxi, came to Durham to help get us settled. Jimmie and I stayed in a beautiful motel on the outskirts of town so our babies would be more comfortable while the moving van was being unloaded. Since there was no room for Mattie in our car, she rode the bus to Durham.

Because of her color, Mattie was refused a room at the motel. We weren't able to talk the owner into allowing her to stay in the motel with us even though she was there to nurse our babies. Instead, Mattie had to stay in a Durham hotel catering to blacks. Although I'd grown up in Louisiana, this was my first experience with how real segregation worked. I was both shocked and surprised.

Having gone to Durham earlier to find a place for us to live, Jimmie had purchased a lovely home on the corner of Kent Street. Set among a lush growth of trees on a gravel road on rolling hills, our home held a special beauty, but our happiness over moving into such a pretty place was soon marred.

Benita Ann was sick again. All the way to Durham, she

screamed with pain. Nothing made her comfortable. If she got in a certain position, she would sleep for short stretches of time. But when we hit a bump in the road, she would turn and scream for what seemed forever. So Jimmie and I drove directly to Duke Hospital and admitted her before even moving into our house.

Here we were once again — in another strange hospital with doctors we didn't know. Jimmie carried Benita Ann into the hospital and up to the ward while I stayed in the car with Jim. After what seemed to be an eternity, Jimmie returned to tell me to go up to see her. There seemed to be no end to what this illness demanded of us. This hospital had the same rules: parents were not allowed to stay with their children. At least this hospital allowed one hour of visiting daily. Because Jimmie was on the house staff, he could visit Benita Ann at any time.

Once more, I had to leave a precious child of mine in the hands of others and go away. I knew that this time, Benita Ann was aware of very little, but she looked very tiny and defenseless in that big bed with only strangers to look after her. For a moment, I felt like I couldn't leave. But as I looked around the ward, I realized I had no choice. She needed help. We had taken her to the best place we knew to get that help, and I had to leave. For me to place her in that bed and leave her again for more testing and observation was heartbreaking. But if the doctors could discover the cause for her screaming, it would surely be worth it.

By the autumn of 1956, Jimmie and I were able to remove the frame on the bottom of Jim's stroller, and Jim was able to use his feet to push himself about. He followed me everywhere as I placed furniture in our new home. Having bedrooms for each of the children was a luxury, and keeping busy kept me from thinking about Benita Ann in the hospital. I wanted so much to be with her, but that was impossible. Jim needed me. It was good my place was with him.

*****

Jimmie began his residency with enthusiasm although his thoughts were always in the pediatric ward. His day at the hospital began at seven in the morning, and he returned home around six in the evening. He had to report for work at seven on Saturday and Sunday, too. On daily hospital rounds, he usually visited Benita Ann and often made quick visits several times a day. His visits and reports eased my mind.

Once again, we were at the mercy of neurosurgeons. One of them, Dr. Odom, was originally from New Orleans and developed a genuine camaraderie with us since we were from that same part of the country. That helped.

Benita Ann was in the hospital for observation and tests for a month before she was taken to the operating room. In the first surgical procedure on August 3, 1956, the ventriculo-cervical shunt in her neck was removed. On August 26, the ventriculo-ureteral shunt was also removed. Obviously, Benita Ann's hydrocephalus was being compensated since the shunts were no longer necessary. She no longer had symptoms of her original condition. No one had any explanation for this.

During Benita Ann's stay at Duke University Hospital, I felt very helpless. Before, I always thought I understood the purpose of the surgeries, but now, without my really knowing why, doctors continued performing more procedures. I really felt they didn't have any answers either.

Benita Ann's only symptom was crying. Her fontanel was normal. She didn't have any symptoms of hydrocephalus. Then on August 31, an exploratory procedure into her mid-brain was performed. We were told this procedure was necessary to cauterize the source of the spinal fluid so her body would cease producing it. But there was no excess fluid!

For each surgical procedure, I'd go over to Duke Hospital and sit in a waiting room to be near Benita Ann. Jimmie, naturally, had to work, but that was a blessing. While I waited alone for this operation to be completed, a neurosurgeon came down to tell me we should consider finding a home for Benita

Ann. He felt she needed good total care because she was no longer aware of the world around her. Two of his arguments were we had one child at home with hydrocephalus who required special care and our new baby was expected any day.

I rebelled completely at this idea, but I understood he was only trying to be helpful. I sat still looking at him, not volunteering my thoughts. I really believe this last operation to cauterize the glands that produce the spinal fluid was unnecessary. I couldn't protest because I didn't have the answers, and Jimmie and I felt we had to go along with what was recommended.

I thought back to before the surgery when the doctor thumped Jim's head and then Benita Ann's and said, "Do you hear the difference?"

There was a difference, but I never did understand what he meant, and he didn't explain.

There was no way I'd take Benita Ann out of Duke and back to Boston while Jimmie worked. Jim needed me at home, and our new baby was due at any time. So I visited Benita Ann each day for as long as allowed. The children's ward had no air conditioning at this time. In spite of the high ceilings, the big open windows, and buzzing fans, it was still a miserably hot place.

Benita Ann was a beautiful baby, making it easier for the nurses to become fond of her. I felt they cared for her with love rather than duty, and we were thankful for this kindness. Surely, her being handled gently and tenderly made a difference.

After Benita Ann's stitches were removed, we were happy she was allowed to come home with us. She still rolled back and forth, making her singing tunes at all hours of the night. When we placed our hands on her stomach and rocked her gently in her bed, she'd giggle. That was about the only response we could muster from her, but I believe our care and love reached her in some way.

*****

As soon as Jimmie and I arrived in Durham, we located a gynecologist because our new baby was due in about two months. During this time, Duke was making special advances in delivery and infant care, so I attended classes to exercise and learn proper breathing techniques to relax during delivery. Each of us expectant mothers visited the labor and delivery rooms to mentally prepare for our deliveries. I was even allowed to try the anesthetic mask I'd administer myself when I felt I needed a whiff to dull the labor pain. I was to place the mask over my nose, and when I had enough anesthesia, the mask would automatically drop away. Although I'd already had two babies, I found these preparations very helpful to relieve my anxieties.

I liked all this extra attention, especially because this was a new doctor and a new hospital. I also liked their new ideas about infant care. Instead of placing babies in the nursery immediately after birth, the babies were given to their mothers for care. According to this rooming-in theory, babies should be held, loved and fed by their mothers right away to offer the security a cold, indifferent nursery wouldn't provide.

*****

Jimmie and I found out what real Southern hospitality was all about when the lady next door invited all our neighborhood to her home to watch the college All-Star game. There we met two couples who befriended us and made our year in North Carolina a joy. They entertained us, introduced us to native Durhamites, and saw that we enjoyed all the city had to offer, even showing us their summer escape from Durham — Myrtle Beach, South Carolina.

During the fall, they drove us through the mountains so we could witness nature's spectacular colors in the autumn leaves. We met their parents, and when our families visited, they also entertained them. I still marvel that people can give so generously of themselves to an unknown couple who needed friendship so desperately.

Our Tarheel friends even helped me find someone to help with all my babies. Emma Norwood was a dear and learned quickly how to properly handle Benita Ann and Jim in anticipation of the time I'd be at the hospital to deliver our new baby. Jim loved people and attention; therefore, he was happy with Emma.

Back in Thibodaux, new cousins were being born regularly. I learned this was standard in a Catholic family. On September 11, 1956, we received a call from Jimmie's sister Bernice saying she had just had a little girl she named Jane. Two other nieces were born that same year, and just two days later, I had our little girl, the fourth girl born in the Peltier family in 1956.

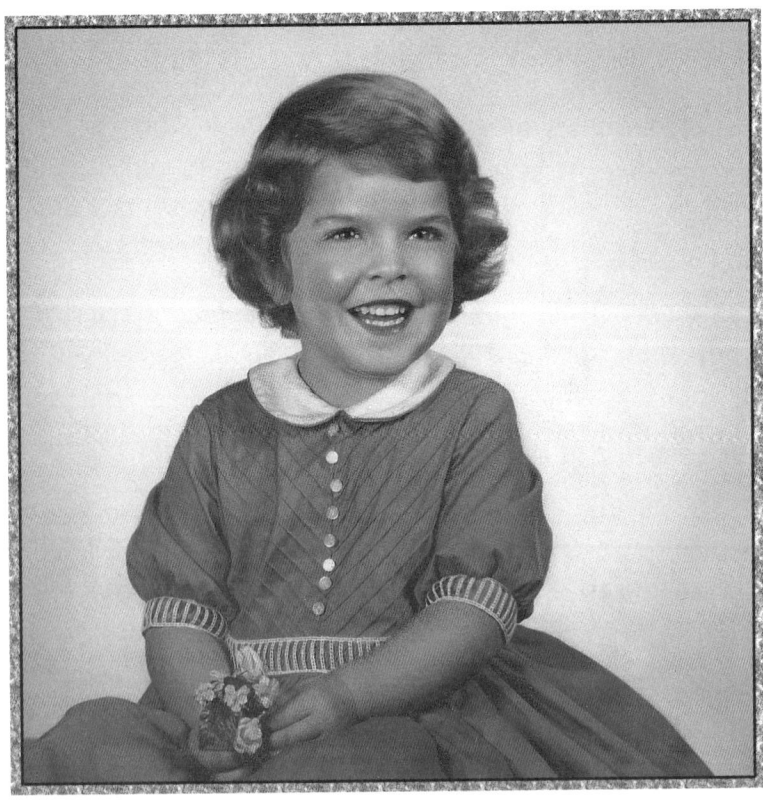

Jeanne Ellen Peltier

When my labor pains began this time, I had trouble waking Jimmie. At first I felt angry because he was moving so slowly, but then I had to laugh when I saw him sitting on the side of the bed half-dressed and sound asleep.

Preparation for delivery made time pass more quickly. With the help of a saddle block, Jeanne Ellen was born at five in the morning on Friday, September 13. She looked different from our other two babies. She had long dark hair, and her skin wasn't as fair. I felt her fontanel. It was normal. But I still was apprehensive because Benita Ann's hydrocephalus didn't manifest itself for three weeks.

Moments after Jeanne Ellen's birth, the neurosurgeons and pediatricians arrived from all over the hospital to check her. Jimmie saw Dr. Odom at a distance in one of the halls holding his hands clasped over his head in a victory gesture. Jeanne was healthy. Our baby was healthy!

After delivery, I was completely exhausted, so the doctors and Jimmie felt I shouldn't follow the rooming-in policy at Duke. Instead, our baby should be placed in the nursery. I felt guilty because she was the only baby in the nursery. All the others were in their mother's rooms. After being reassured that Jeanne had four nurses full time, I lay back waiting for the time to pass to confirm she was healthy. **And she was!** Her fontanel remained like that of other babies, slightly sunken in between the head bones with a normal pulsating heartbeat.

I felt a joy, a happiness I find hard to describe. I suppose it was a feeling of rightness with the world — security for the future — a feeling I could talk with people about Jeanne. Before I didn't want to say much about my two babies because I knew I made others feel sad or at a loss for words, and I didn't like making anyone uncomfortable.

Now I hated to go to sleep at night because I liked imagining how much fun caring for Jeanne would be — all the little normal everyday things other mothers and fathers do with their babies, we could now do with Jeanne. I'd wept over finding out our first two children were sick, now I soaked up the happiness and was thankful to God. In fact, I found myself saying to God, "Isn't this nicer? Surely, you must enjoy this more than pain and sadness!"

But most of all, I loved seeing Jimmie smiling and happy. He couldn't have been a prouder father. His walk had a special spring, and when he came home from the hospital in his green surgery scrubs, we didn't have to say what we felt; we just looked into each other's eyes and knew. We'd grown up together these past two and a half years; now we lived this new joy intensely.

When offering to God each day my joys and my sorrows, it was great to have this keenly felt joy to give to Him. Jimmie and I both thanked Him endlessly.

Having a baby had always been a miracle to me. Now having a healthy baby was an even greater miracle. To this day, as they did then, my thoughts go back to that letter from Pope Pius XII saying he'd pray for our baby.

Presents, cards, telegrams, flowers poured from our family and friends.

My mother, always there when I needed her, arrived the morning following Jeanne's birth to help with Jim and Benita Ann while I was confined to the hospital. I loved seeing the glow on her face as she gazed at her new grandchild.

My mother was alone with Jim and Benita Ann only from six-thirty in the morning when Jimmie left for work until nine in the morning when Emma arrived. But with two sick children, even that short amount of time was frightening. One morning she called me at seven o'clock saying Jim and Benita Ann were both crying. I told her what to do — put Jim on the floor with his bicycle upside down, turn the wheel, and turn Benita Ann's music box on — and they hushed.

In Protestant Durham, St. Mary Magdalene Church was almost considered mission land because of the small number of Catholics. So Catholics worked harder and tried with more enthusiasm to do what they could for the church. Jimmie and I had come to know Father Joseph Klaus well, so he baptized

Jeanne at St. Mary Magdalene in September 1956.

Since Jeanne's godparents were from Thibodaux, they were unable to attend; however, she had full baptismal rites, followed by a toast of champagne at our home. As Father Klaus, Jimmie and I lifted our glasses and touched them together, we were very happy.

The next few months were busy and happy for us. Jim was going everywhere in his stroller; Benita Ann enjoyed lying in her bed or in a buggy; and Jeanne was growing like a normal baby.

Jeanne was beautiful. She looked like the baby in the Gerber advertisement, only prettier. When I played with her, she felt like a little round ball. Just to handle her was a pleasure because Jeanne had strength in her neck. No special care was needed to support her head and body as had been the case with our two other children. Handling a normal baby was fun. Jim liked our new addition, and I loved the everydayness of it all.

One day while Benita Ann and Jeanne were sleeping, I received a telephone call from my elderly friend who lived next door with her daughter and son-in-law. "Please come quickly. My daughter does not seem well!" were her words.

Having had troubles of my own, I was more than willing to help, so I took Jim into my arms and hurried over. When we got there, she met me at the door saying, "Hurry! Down here in the basement!"

We went down the stairs. There was her daughter, hanging from a rope tied to a rafter. Her face was blue, and her tongue was protruding. Suicide!

I wanted to run out of there, but I offered to call somebody. My neighbor, however, insisted we cut her daughter down first to save her life, although I knew she was dead. I put Jim down on the floor, helped her cut the rope, and we lowered her daughter's body to the floor. I had to muster all the courage and strength I had in me to cut that rope because the old woman wanted this done so desperately. I had few intelligent thoughts by now, so I called Jimmie at Duke for help.

Jimmie was in surgery. All he could say was for me to call the police. I should have known to do that without being told, but I was having trouble gathering my thoughts. All this time, Jim had been jabbering to himself and pointing at all going on. I was relieved when the police arrived and assumed command. I could honestly tell the police I had to rush back to see about my other two children. Once again, I realized how we are often powerless to help others.

*****

Birth control was a continuing problem for Jimmie and me. We had previously tried the rhythm method, my having to count eight days after my monthly period and our having to abstain from sexual intercourse for the next ten days. But we learned that because of our traumatic upsets from our children's hospital admissions, I couldn't count on a regular ovulation time. So we began using the temperature method, which required my recording on detailed, elaborate charts my daily morning temperature. When a slight drop in my temperature indicated ovulation, we then needed to abstain from sexual intercourse, not easy for a twenty-six year old couple very much in love.

Jimmie and I had never considered artificial means of birth control, and I'm sure many people thought we were foolish. Maybe we were, but the Catholic Church said "no," and we obeyed what we had been told. Jimmie had always been committed to following Catholic Church rules. Since I was now a Catholic, the thought of breaking the rules never entered our minds. We had wanted a nice-sized family. We could afford to care for our children. But after our having two hydrocephalic children who required so much of our time and attention and caused us a great deal of worry, we really didn't want to keep having children. So we conscientiously placed this phase of our life in God's hands.

*****

I enjoyed buying clothes for our three babies. Our friends in Durham also had young children, so they often invited me to ride with them to Chapel Hill and once even to Raleigh to shop for our children. These trips would take an hour or two and were wonderful fun for me. Because the children were all doing well and I had good help, I took advantage of these short trips away from the house. I knew I should go when the opportunities were offered because I simply needed a respite, but I was surprised these short excursions of mine were good for our children, too. They needed time away from Mother, too.

Jim ate well and was a happy person. Now he was able to hold his head up and could use a regular high chair, which offered him another diversion during his waking day. He often said, "Floor," because that was a change from the stroller for him. Because he couldn't walk or play outside, he didn't get dirty.

Jim was my best friend. He went everywhere with me. In the early days when I didn't know anybody and didn't even know my way around Durham, the two of us went exploring each day. With Jim sitting beside me, I ventured farther and farther from Kent Street until I had learned what I could about our new hometown from the window of our car. Before long, I knew the city as well as the natives.

And in his special way, so did Jim. Once when my aunt and uncle were visiting, Jim guided them home across town merely by what he could see from his low vantage point in the middle of the front seat. They marveled that he could look at tree tops and give directions at only two and a half years of age.

Sometimes the pressure from the cerebral fluid stimulates a child's brain, making the child unusually bright. I don't know if that was the case with Jim or not, but he and I talked all the time and enjoyed each other's company. Of course, he was a captive audience. Because he couldn't walk and I always moved him from room to room with me, he was rarely alone. The only time I was out of his sight was when he was absorbed in a TV show. Then I could say to him, "I'm going to the kitchen to wash dishes, and I'll be right back."

I always told Jim the truth, and he learned he could depend on what I said. He had a good sense of humor, and I felt lucky to have such a true best friend. I liked the time of day that allowed me to give him my total attention, especially during baths and meals. He was understanding about Benita Ann and called her "Me Ann." I have always thought of myself as a quiet person, but I kept up a steady chatter with Jim as we spent a lot of time growing mentally and spiritually.

Jim and his daddy also had a great rapport. Jimmie has always been very popular with children, and with Jim's brightness and his sensitivity to people, the two of them spent many good times together.

Jim laughed and responded in such a way that he dominated situations, charmed adults, and helped everyone feel special.

Jim had beautiful skin. I was amused by the mole on top of his foot right near his little toe like the one I had in exactly the same place. When he lifted his arms to be picked up, I loved putting my hands under his arms and feeling his cheek next to mine. That year I tried spending as much time with him as possible in the fresh air enjoying the wonderful weather in Durham.

*****

When Jimmie had first arrived in Durham, he had looked for an apartment or a house to rent, but none were available. With two sick children and a baby due a month after we arrived, his buying a home seemed logical, so he did. Our ability to do this seemed to bother a goodly number of other residents and interns.

This resentment didn't affect my life as much as it did Jimmie's. One of his supervisors in the oral surgery service deliberately decided to make this year difficult and almost unbearable for Jimmie. That is when all of the wonderful traits I love and admire in Jimmie came to the forefront.

The badgering began on hospital rounds early every Sunday morning. All the oral and plastic surgery residents made grand rounds together. Jimmie, as the latest addition to the group, was often quizzed unmercifully by the chief. After one such terrible morning, out came the books from the library. Jimmie began long hours of extra study each night that eventually helped him endure the Sunday morning quizzes. Each Saturday, he would go over every patient's chart, reading everything he could about each particular surgical problem so he'd be prepared to answer the chief's questions on Sunday. As traumatic as this experience was and as humiliating as the hammering questions were, Jimmie became a better person and a better oral surgeon for having endured this difficult time and for never having had a weekend off during that entire year.

Our new Durham friends helped us through this by sharing Saturday nights with Jimmie and me. We barbecued or ate at the nice restaurants in the area. Jimmie and I looked forward to that one night of relaxation each week. I don't know what we would have done without our friends!

The Durham church people were very friendly and enthusiastic, and I joined their ladies' organization. When plans were being made for a fund-raising luncheon, I offered to make chicken-a-la-king for three hundred people. I borrowed electric ovens and plugged them up and down the hall. As I made small batches of the mixture, I emptied them into pans and put the pans in the ovens. It took two days, but sure enough, I got it all made as well as the toast cups. I believe I surprised the Catholic ladies; I know I surprised myself.

Family members came to visit us as much as possible. I made little scrapbooks to show Jim pictures of our family so he could say their names and be familiar with everyone when we'd return to Louisiana.

Christmas came, and we loved preparing our own turkey

and dressing and being Santa Claus in our own home. We were happy to be well, and we enjoyed our day even though we were missing our family's big celebration back in Louisiana.

Our pediatrician suggested we take Jim to Children's Hospital for physical therapy to help strengthen his legs. When we took him into the therapy room, they worked with him on ramps built with railings to support him as he practiced walking. Jim liked people and wanted attention.

One day a small fund-raising bazaar was held in the hospital parking lot. All the handicapped patients and their parents participated. As Jimmie and I stood there, we noticed the visible parents' love as they watched their children enjoy ordinary activities routine for normal children.

As the sun shone and the rain began to fall at the same time, Jimmie looked at me saying, "This weather is just like the scene in front of us. The sun represents the parents with love and hope for their happy children and such joy at seeing them having fun. When you look closer and notice the handicaps their children have, it is as if the rains falls to mar the brightness."

*****

Though Jimmie was receiving great academic training at Duke, he realized he'd get further training and more surgical experience at Charity Hospital in New Orleans. He felt the combination of the two programs would better prepare him for oral surgery. After giving the matter much thought, he applied to Charity and was accepted into their program. Charity Hospital's medical director was an old friend from Thibodaux, Dr. Leo Kerne. Many years before, Dr. Kerne had taken Jimmie into the operating room to observe surgery. It would be a great reunion, and we were happy knowing we would be going back to Louisiana in a few months.

Chapter Eleven

Much Hope Again

In February, I realized I was expecting again. The miserable nausea started once again, and Jimmie's days were even longer. He willingly got up early each morning to change our three babies' dirty morning diapers before he left for work. His help was unbelievable in preventing me from getting sick before I could feed our children breakfast. I wondered how many fathers would do such an unpleasant job at five o'clock in the morning to show their love.

One afternoon shortly before we packed to leave Durham, Jim was in his stroller in my bedroom and pushed the button on the doorknob, locking himself in. Because our house was built on a hill, I was unable to crawl through the windows to unlock the door. I talked to Jim through the door to keep him calm and tried telling him to turn the doorknob to open the door, but to no avail.

Across the street from us was the back gate to the home of the famous Mrs. Angie Biddle Duke. Each day, seven servants arrived and departed through that locked gate. Just when I realized I wouldn't be able to get Jim out alone, I remembered it was time for these men to end their day.

Only too happy to help. all seven came in and removed the whole door from its hinges to get Jim out. They seemed to enjoy the change from their routine as they accepted my thanks.

Before we left Durham, Jimmie and I hosted a party for all who'd befriended us during this year and we'd come to love, eternally grateful for the way all of them shared their lives with us and made us a part of a community while we were away from home. Their friendship was a treasure.

Because traveling back to Louisiana was no easy job, Jimmie and I decided traveling by train would be the best way to return. Both our mothers came to Durham to help our three children and me make the trip. Benita Ann required a comfortable spot on which to lie so she'd be touched and handled as little as possible. Jim needed constant entertaining because he'd have to remain sitting, and I was the only one strong enough to carry him everywhere. Jeanne was nine months old and easy to handle, but her being a baby on a train for two nights and three days also required someone to take care of her.

We were a strange sight — three women, one of whom was pregnant, and three babies. We three were carrying all the bottles two babies would need and enough diapers for all three of my babies.

When we arrived in New Orleans, Mrs. Peltier stayed in our motel room on Airline Highway with my three babies while my mother and I went to get the key to the new house which Jimmie and I had purchased from our old friend, Hank Lauricella.

Jimmie met Hank when they were young boys playing on Grand Isle, and their friendship had been renewed as college students. Hank was an All American who played football for the University of Tennessee. His wife Betsy and I had become close friends after the Lauricellas moved to New Orleans. Hank was now in the real estate business, so it was natural for us to call on him to find a house. After getting the keys from Hank and looking at the house, I contacted the moving van and moved into yet another house.

Jimmie and I had just ended one of the happiest years of our life. We hadn't been in a hospital for ten months,

AND we had a healthy baby! Well aware of our blessings, we thanked God.

*****

As Hurricane Audrey was gaining strength in the Gulf of Mexico for its devastating entry into Cameron, Louisiana, we were putting three baby beds together and moving into 5912 Camphor Street, just outside of New Orleans. Airline Park in Metairie was one of the early subdivisions built on reclaimed marshland. Since Jimmie needed to be able to make a quick run to Charity Hospital, we thought we'd made a good choice. Of course, we found out he'd need forty-five minutes for that quick run during busy traffic hours. Having grown up in small towns, this seemed like a waste of time. Even at Duke, Jimmie was just a few minutes away from the hospital.

I'd always fallen in love with each home we moved into, no matter how it looked. Our new pre-fabricated house on the back row of Airline Park with a swamp for a front yard was beautiful because Jimmie shared it with me. With three children and a fourth arriving shortly, I found myself again being very hopeful and optimistic about the future.

Jimmie and I had become spoiled by our few months' absence from hospitals. How quickly we could put the unpleasantness out of our thoughts was surprising.

Up until we left Durham, the doctors at Duke continued to insist we put Benita Ann into a home. As a favor to the two of us, some had even written letters to Louisiana in search of homes that would provide her total care. Very few residential homes for mentally handicapped children would accept patients needing total care. Most preferred physically handicapped children who could be educated to some extent.

Occasionally, a facility would take a totally dependent child under eighteen, but not often. One such home had just been built by Bishop Charles P. Greco in the central Louisiana Diocese of Alexandria. It offered something directed toward our needs, but we filed the papers away hoping we could forget about having to use them. Though I was willing to hear these discussions, I hadn't for a minute seriously thought about making the decision to go through with such a plan for Benita Ann.

Both Jimmie and I had occasional anxieties about the new baby we were expecting, but we both had abiding faith in God. We continued attending daily Mass whenever possible, and we prayed in our own private way many times daily. Jeanne was normal in every way, and we assumed all would be well. Having so little time to think of ourselves was really a blessing.

Charity Hospital provided Jimmie with so much of every phase of oral surgery for him to perform that he quickly found a niche for himself. This program didn't require the long days on duty every weekend required at Duke, so having him at home so much more was a luxury. Just as he'd been considerate those first months during my nausea, he was still helpful with our babies. He changed diapers or did menial tasks for each of them as readily as I did and helped prepare them for bed each night. We usually put the children to sleep by six o'clock in the evening so we could share long evenings together.

*****

Shortly after getting settled on Camphor Street, Jim and I went exploring. Once when I was walking with him among toys in a store, he spotted a tricycle in the shape of a missile and fell in love with it. Much to his surprise and mine, he could reach the pedals and move them. How wonderful! Another way he could get around and be outside to talk and play with other children.

This tricycle was a special toy that was not only imaginative, but also offered more balance than a regular tricycle. Tears came to my eyes with the bursting pride I felt as I stood in the driveway watching Jim pedal about. At first, he went slowly down the driveway to the sidewalk. Then the freedom this missile represented seemed to dawn on him.

A whole new world opened for Jim that day. When he was on his missile, he became like all the other children as they met each morning to explore the world. This was a world others took for granted, but when Jim pedaled on the sidewalk, he really was having a first look at a brave new world. The days weren't long enough for him now. When we tucked him in and said his prayers with him each night, I felt even God had no idea He'd receive such thanks for a small thing like a missile tricycle.

When Jeanne began to walk, Jim was more pleased than anyone else. Whenever someone came to the house, he'd say, "Jeanne can walk!"

I'd have been heartbroken at his words had I felt he realized he was different and couldn't walk, but this wasn't in his thoughts at all. His world was perfectly secure. He accepted it as it was. He had all the love and attention he wanted. We ran when he called. Our legs were his legs to move at his will. He was proud of Jeanne. He simply loved his sister and was happy when she learned to do something new. He also had someone new to wait on him because he ordered her about just as he did the rest of us.

Our home was so new it had no lawn, just dirt and a few weeds. As we spent late evening hours outside sprigging St. Augustine grass and pulling weeds, Jim rode his missile; Benita Ann lay in her buggy; and Jeanne played in the dirt. Who would think seeing their baby girl in the dirt could give a mother and father any special good feelings? Becoming more aware of moments like these, I often just closed my eyes and said, "Thank you, God." But moments like these weren't lasting.

One day while visiting some of our friends, Jim tried to sit on a friend's tricycle and fell on the cement. Because of his enlarged head, Jim's head naturally hit first and with more force. He cried the usual tears and was comforted fairly easily. However, we weren't comforted. We knew; we watched; we hoped. Soon we knew we were in trouble as Jim began to become drowsy and then to vomit.

Having been discharged from the Navy, Dr. Garcia was back in New Orleans, so we met him at the familiar Mercy Hospital emergency room. Instead of another flare up of hydrocephalic pressure, Jim had a brain concussion and went into a deep sleep. I packed again, moved into Room 516, and sat by his bed, watching, hoping he would move, hoping he would wake up. Jim slept for five days.

Whenever we moved into a new town, I had to employ reliable help right away because we didn't know when I would have to be in the hospital with one of our children. Though our families weren't distant in miles, they had always been too far away to know how to handle our children and to feel comfortable doing so. They felt a certain fear because of the hydrocephalus, and we understood their feelings. Teaching an available, trustworthy person the routine and having her call if there were any unexpected troubles was always better. Being so willing and loving to share the chores with me, Flora Cohn stayed with Benita Ann and Jeanne during the day, as Jimmie, their very capable, giving father, took night duty.

*****

Jim was beautiful as he lay there asleep. Dr. Garcia was sure time would bring him around. As I watched Jim, I remembered his past surgeries and became all too aware he was growing taller and that the tube from his head to his ureter would have to be replaced. In 1955 that first ventriculo-ureteral shunt had been revised and lengthened after just six months. Even though Jim had had no symptoms, the doctors in Boston felt that a certain number of inches growth was sufficient reason to change the tubing.

Two years had passed since the last revision. Jim had grown several inches; however, the doctor said the surgeons left extra length in the tubing to allow for his growth. Both the doctors in Durham and Dr. Garcia wanted to leave well enough alone, never knowing but always hoping Jim might compensate for hydrocephalus and be cured. Dr. Garcia knew we watched Jim very closely and would immediately report anything out of the ordinary.

I thought and wondered again about Jim's legs and why he couldn't walk. He had a gorgeous little boy's body with beautifully shaped legs. Only his slightly enlarged head covered with a soft mop of blonde hair suggested an abnormality, but he had a bright, happy personality.

For the first ten months of his life, Jim's head had continued to grow. He had suffered many episodes of increased pressure and had experienced many taps to remove the excess fluid. His enlarged head made it difficult for him to balance and learn to walk. The many hours of increased intracranial pressure had weakened his legs. But from 1955 to 1957, he had grown stronger while his hydrocephalus had stabilized.

Jim had no fear of doctors. During this hospital admission, just as in all the earlier ones, I held Jim close to me for the necessary injections. I had learned from all the hours and minutes together just what could entertain him and distract his thoughts, and I would have gone to any length to lessen any pain.

At last, Jim opened his eyes — those beautiful, light green, sparkling eyes with a twinkle like his father's. My best friend was back with me! He was hungry, and all the nurses on the floor got him anything he wanted at any hour, especially Mrs. McCarthy, the same kind head nurse, and Sister Marie Jeanne, the nun who had been born in Thibodaux. Jim had spent three months of his first year on the fifth floor with them, so they felt he was partly their baby.

Everyone knew Jim had returned to normal when we found ourselves once again jumping at his every command. He wanted to go home, and when he told the doctor he was ready, we were discharged. The next day, back to the missile tricycle he went. His fall had been a freak occurrence, and we couldn't deny him this pleasure.

Jimmie had had a busy time back on Camphor Street

during our absence. My being in the hospital with Jim all those worrisome days was hard, but I feel sure Jimmie's role was more difficult. It's worse to be away from the sick one you love, worrying at a distance about what is going on in the sick room, than to be there physically with the sick person you're helping.

Chapter Twelve

Annette - Our Fourth Child

*T*ime arrived to buy another baby bed. That we needed four baby beds seemed unreal. But our new baby would arrive in October. Before I knew it, it was October.

As it so often seemed to happen, my labor began during the night. The long train I'd hoped wouldn't block our rush to Baptist Hospital was, indeed, stopped across the track on Airline Highway. We were exasperated, but the caboose finally came into sight, and we arrived at the hospital in time. I was prepped and given the spinal anesthetic. This time Jimmie was present to witness his first delivery, and we shared the joy of the birth of our fourth child. Another baby girl was born to Ann and Jimmie Peltier on October 9, 1957. All of us in the delivery room were trying to be the first to touch her fontanel. It felt normal, soft, and slightly sunken.

With no sleep, Jimmie reported to Charity Hospital that morning with "It's a girl!" cigars.

In that four-bed ward, my corner of privacy with my own thoughts was a haven for me. My baby was brought to me about noon, and she was fine. The pediatrician had checked her, and Jimmie and his fellow residents visited us about six in the evening. We felt such jubilation for our new baby girl that we decided to name her Annette Marie – Annette after me and Marie after the Blessed Mother.

I was still working on my devotion to Mary, the Mother of God. Not having been reared in the Catholic faith and not having developed this love for Mary as a child, I couldn't readily accept something so foreign to me. I'd been reading everything I could about Mary. Using her name for one of my children seemed to be another step in my learning to appreciate her as so many Catholics do.

When Annette was brought to me again at around eight that evening, I noted a change in her fontanel only thirteen hours after her birth. While holding my beautiful little baby — that tiny, innocent, unknowing little baby and looking down at her, all those hours of suffering that Jim and Benita Ann had experienced came flooding back. I felt the two of us were

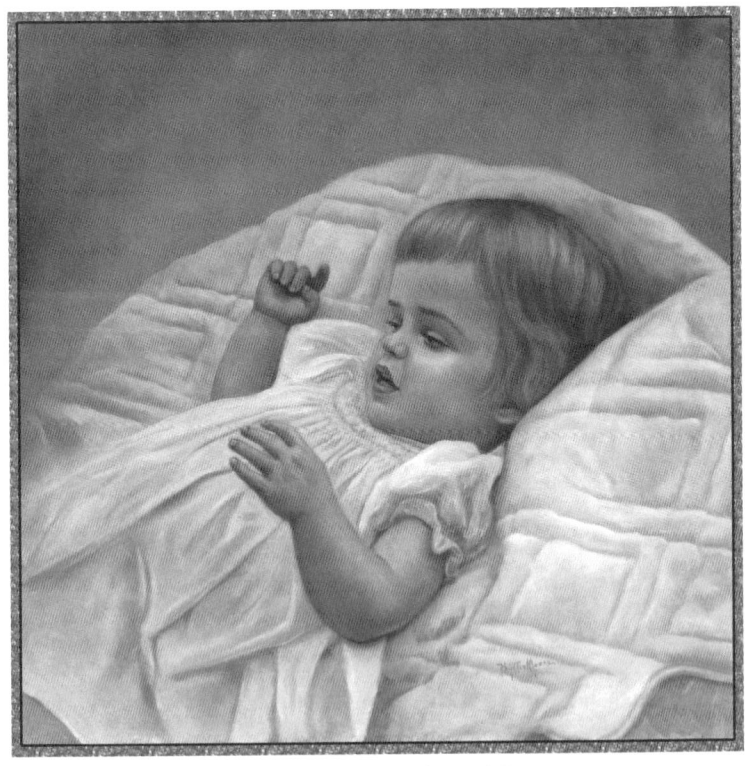

Annette Marie Peltier

very alone. This time I felt God had forsaken us. The question of "why" could no longer be repressed. I wondered where He was; was there really a God? If so, He must not care much for my family.

I didn't want to hand Annette to the nurse to be taken back into the nursery. I wanted time to stand still for Annette and me. I would have liked for things to remain static, to stop the slow filling up of her fontanel I knew too well each hour would bring. The nurse didn't take her away.

I lay back in my bed and looked at the cornice over the drapes, seeing a clear picture in my mind of a field of grass about knee-high, the wind blowing slightly, and me running away across the field. Then, very clearly, I felt a presence and heard the sentence, "Ann, you cannot run. She has hydrocephalus, and you have to face it."

I felt very calm, but I also felt a great hurt, a hurt impossible to describe — a heavy weight inside, and, yet, no tears. Had our children been stillborn, or maybe never born, would have been easier. I kept thinking in my bitter despair, *God is so clever to give us children with that deforming condition*; yet I kept holding every hope that if the surgery could correct it, they could live normal lives.

After a time, I got up and walked far down the long hall to call Dr. Garcia on the pay telephone. I felt if I could tell him, maybe he could start procedures sooner so Annette's head wouldn't grow too large. He responded in his usual cool, professional manner. I realized my call wouldn't rush him. He'd wait for her to grow before he'd operate, but I felt better just telling him of the situation. I'd accepted the truth and was ready to face it.

I was moved to a private room. Beautiful, over-full bouquets of flowers began to arrive — flowers perfect in their glorious colors and grandeur, but down the hall somewhere in the nursery was a tiny little girl with an even tinier imperfection that wasn't allowing spinal fluid to escape from her head. There seemed to be a flaw in life's plan.

I don't know when the phrase *I am not going to think about it* took its place in my repertoire, but I feel perhaps it was now. I wore the beautiful gowns and robes friends and family sent and ate the delicious food as the hours passed until Annette and I could return home.

Time wasn't going to stop for us. We'd have to proceed down that long, winding path again, a path different for each child, but one filled with pain and heartaches for us all. I don't feel I showed my friends how completely dejected I really was. What good would that do? One friend even came and brought a lovely lace bonnet. I'm sure she never realized that tiny little hat was made for babies with beautifully shaped heads and that we'd have no use for it.

During each of our children's illnesses, it was as though Jimmie, our child, and I all had hydrocephalus. He and I would take every step our child took. It would be the same for Annette. There would never be moments when thoughts of her didn't fill our minds. Yet she'd have to lie in that big hospital baby bed alone. She'd face the tests and examinations alone. If only we could have had hydrocephalus instead of her. But *I am not going to think about it* ran through my mind. Sometimes I'd just say that sentence over and over and over until I couldn't think; I was just numb.

In the past when I realized my child had hydrocephalus, I felt sorrow not only for our child, Jimmie and me, but for others whose lives were touched. This time I felt differently. I had no such kind thoughts about others. Jimmie and I were older; we had large, serious troubles; and I had to struggle to handle my own thoughts. I somehow felt Jimmie was also going through the same feelings.

Jimmie and I now knew what we had to steel ourselves for, and we were individually trying to reach for courage. No longer was there anything anyone could say or do to help us at this point.

We wanted no domestic help at night; instead, we just wanted to pull the four walls of the house around us and have all six of us together to share what sleeping hours we could. Having a new baby with hydrocephalus made real the need for Benita Ann to go away to live in a total care environment. As that reality begin to take shape somewhere in the backs of our minds, I pushed it away saying, *I am not going to think about it!*

One night Jimmie asked me to get the Bible out and read from Job. Job had experienced such devastation in his life. I hoped I could continue to say "Thy will be done" as Job had. Actually, I'd stopped asking God for help — I really had turned everything over to Him. Why not? All my asking didn't seem to matter anyway.

Because Benita Ann had started screaming again whenever she was touched, Dr. Garcia decided to admit her and Annette into the hospital at the same time on October 16, 1957. No double room was available, so the girls were placed at opposite ends of Mercy Hospital's fifth floor.

Jimmie later told me about one of the terrible moments he'd never forget. When he stepped off the elevator into the hospital corridor on the fifth floor, he heard two babies crying — one coming from the left down the hall and the other from the right. He suddenly realized both cries came from his little girls as a picture of each lying in her hospital bed was clear in his mind. How could he choose which to visit first to offer help, help he knew could bring no lasting comfort? Having to do something, he just turned to the right.

*****

Finally, we were able to get a double room with private duty nurses around the clock. I still needed to be with my two sick children all day because they demanded more than two hands can manage. Their room was very depressing — in one bed was tiny Annette, our infant who, at first glance, seemed to be in perfect health. In the other bed was Benita Ann, our baby with the same disease, but a baby with an enlarged head who was blind and mentally handicapped.

Jimmie and I had tried very hard to have hope for Annette. I never entered my daughter's room without marveling at my ability to do so without tears. I often wondered if I was a hard, unfeeling person. I did what I didn't think myself capable of doing — I actually held my head up, smiled, and assisted in making our children comfortable. I don't even remember collapsing into tears in anyone's presence. I don't remember ever running from what was expected of me as a mother. I'm a softhearted person who cries for the *Star Spangled Banner,* a line in a moving piece of poetry, or a sad story about another's illness. So I was surprised I was able to care so calmly for my sick children, doing my duty better than I knew how.

Dr. Menville, a urologist, performed Benita Ann's surgery with Dr. Garcia's assistance. After cystoscoping her, they traced her pain and screaming to the area around her ureter and knew the tube in her ureter wasn't functioning and must be removed. When they did exploratory surgery on October 29, they found the end of the ventriculo-ureteral shunt abscessed because the end that had been anchored in the lower portion of the ureter hadn't been removed when the rest of the tubing was removed in Boston.

That abscess had caused Benita Ann's terrible pain and screaming for eighteen months! The only reason she had been comfortable at all was because we had learned how to handle her gently. Once the anchored end of the tubing was removed, Benita Ann never screamed again.

Because he knew the results would be the same as for our other two children, Dr. Garcia didn't even run preliminary tests like the pneumoencephalogram to determine the location of Annette's blockage. He performed surgery on Annette on November 4 when she wasn't yet a month old.

Up went our hopes again — maybe the shunt would work. Since Annette's head wasn't too large yet, maybe she could be just like a normal baby.

Because she was so tiny, Annette's operation took nine hours. Dr. Garcia tried the Torkildson, a shunt that held such promise if it would only work. Because the neck's growth is so slight, placing the tubing for a short distance in Annette's neck would bypass the existing blockage. If it would begin to function, it could function indefinitely. This would be the ideal answer.

We had been in the hospital when Dr. Garcia had performed the surgery on a little boy. It had worked immediately, and the child had been allowed to go home after only two weeks — and it had continued to work. So of course, we had hope!

Annette came through the surgery beautifully. Like our other two children, she was in perfect health otherwise, and we were thankful.

Because the Torkildson seemed to be working on Annette and Benita Ann was recovering well from the urological surgery, both were discharged on November 23 after a six-week stay in the hospital.

Once again, the six of us shared the same house. It was already the end of November, and Christmas was just around the corner. Since we gave presents to all of our nieces and nephews, I had an unbelievable Christmas list. The belief that the more you have to do, the more you get done is true. I shopped for everybody and even put up a Christmas tree.

Everybody was well, so we had a beautiful Christmas! Holidays are no different from any other day when four dependent babies need to be bathed and fed, but celebrating Jesus's birthday is always something special. I led our children in singing *Happy Birthday, Jesus*, but my thoughts were more on what the Blessed Mother must have felt when she took her baby to be circumcised and St. Simon told her about the future suffering her baby would have to endure. I could now identify with a part of Mary's life and prayed for the courage to be as brave as her.

Chapter Thirteen

Even More Heartbreak

*T*he luxury of a healthy household was quickly over. Annette's Torkildson shunt began to malfunction, so back to the hospital we went. Annette was now three months old, and because her first surgery failed, her head had grown considerably in size. This time, I tried to leave for the hospital without thinking. We had to bring our baby to the hospital; we had to wait for another eight hour surgery; and then we had to wait again to see if the shunt would function properly.

On January 3, Dr. Garcia performed a ventriculo-peritoneal shunt, a new procedure for us. He would run a tube from Annette's mid-brain, where the spinal fluid is produced, out of her head to beneath the skin in the back of her neck. The tube then went down her back into her stomach, where the fluid would then be absorbed.

During this time, I felt like a robot. Maybe living my life as a robot would be the answer because I felt so tired from being up night and day. I needed to move through each day without letting my sensitive mind think. I accomplished no goals while those depressing thoughts constantly nagged at me. I helped no one by feeling angry about our situation.

After Annette had been in the hospital three weeks, she was well enough to go home — certainly a record up until now. The pediatricians were suggesting and now insisting we place Benita Ann in a home. Jimmie began to realize this would be the best course of action now that Annette, too, was sick and her own future was uncertain. Jimmie knew there would be more surgeries for Benita Ann, and he felt Jim's life would be more normal if he didn't have to watch his sister suffer every day.

All those explanations didn't convince me. I could feel wheels bigger than me in motion. I knew we were nearing the day when a decision would have to be made to place Benita Ann in another's care. I felt limp from all that had happened to us and didn't have a valid argument on my side. Sometimes a person has to accept the judgment of people who know more than they.

*****

Clarks lies in the northeast Louisiana piney woods. Years ago, it was a lumber town. After all the available lumber had been depleted and the town had become deserted, Bishop Greco purchased the old hotel and several abandoned houses for use as a home for exceptional children. Through his many contacts in Italy, he employed an order of nuns to staff these quaint quarters and prepare a comfortable place for children needing special care.

Jimmie and I had never before visited a school for mentally handicapped children. Here were the bedridden, the totally mentally handicapped, the elderly mentally handicapped, the mongoloids, and the physically handicapped with mental retardation.

Having swallowed hard at what we saw, we also noticed something refreshing — love and happiness. People spoke softly. Each helpful act was done with loving care and compassion. Over the door to the main entrance, a sign read, "Every child has the right to happiness, but even more so, those who have a more difficult time to earn it."

On this visit, we met Sister Zita, the Directress, and Sister Mary and then drove back to New Orleans, digesting all we had seen as we discussed our day.

Even though the symptoms of Benita Ann's hyrdrocephalus were arrested, she was blind and hardly knew or understood anything. She needed to be fed, bathed, and have her diapers changed. She needed kindness and love, but she had no way of knowing who gave it to her. She'd never know who was caring for her. She didn't know me from anyone else. By thinking this way, I came to terms with the difficult decision of placing her in a foreign environment.

After our having prayed over this huge decision, the day for Benita Ann's departure from our home arrived. Jimmie and I went through the motions without letting ourselves think.

My parents met us in Alexandria, Louisiana, and I felt worse for my mother than anyone. Jimmie and I had wrestled with this decision about Benita Ann and had come to terms with it. But my mother had gotten caught up in something over which she had no control. I know it broke her heart probably more than mine.

Jimmie and I visited Clarks many times after that, always consoled at finding Benita Ann in dry diapers with no plastic covering at any hour of the day or night. When I watched mothers and fathers recognized by their little ones and saw their children run to hug them, crying when they left, I was thankful Benita Ann didn't know us. I was shocked for what I had come to be thankful.

On Camphor Street, there were now only five of us when we turned out the lights at night and said our prayers. Of the five, only Jimmie and I were really aware that one of us was missing, so that was a comfort in a small way.

Long nights of sexual abstinence began. We couldn't have another baby. With three of our four children having hydrocephalus, our odds of having a healthy child weren't good. So I went back to those hallowed halls at Loyola to talk to Father Atherton, his being far removed from our cold reality.

In the quiet beauty of his paneled office, a discussion about abstaining certain days each month sounded simple. But in the dark nights Jimmie and I shared together trying to find some solace from our long worried days, we didn't find those ideals so easy to emulate. Because we never considered artificial birth control, I was still taking my temperature every morning and keeping a graphic chart. Even after all of our troubles, we still had a truly trusting relationship with God and the Catholic Church.

*****

One day, Jim had a common cold, which was unusual around our house. Our family seldom had ordinary illnesses. We seemed to have a special dispensation. However, Jim getting a cold was anything but common, so we had to admit him to Mercy Hospital in February because of his fever and sore throat. He developed some changes with his eyes; otherwise, everything was going smoothly.

While we'd been in Durham, Jim entered the Children's Hospital's physical therapy program to strengthen his legs. After we settled in New Orleans, we began those exercise sessions again as I took him for a forty-five minute drive all the way across New Orleans two or three times weekly. Once Annette was born and needed us during her critical periods, we hired the Metairie Cab Company to come for Jim twice a week to take him to the center. The company was kind enough to send the same driver each time so Jim would feel secure with him, but there were times when Jim was reluctant to go alone. On those days, I watched with a heavy heart as the taxi backed out our driveway. Jim would stand on the floor of the back seat, holding on to the front seat for those trips. Sending him off alone was something else I'd added to my long list of things I had to do.

By now, we had a swing set in our backyard. Jim didn't have the balance to sit on an ordinary swing, but this one was constructed a little like a seesaw. The two seats faced each other with a handle to grasp in the middle, which was perfect for him.

Jim also liked playing in the sandbox, so I encouraged him

to get dirty and know the feel of sand between his fingers and toes. Jeanne, of course, was right in the middle of everything Jim was late in learning to do.

When we realized Jim should be making more progress with his walking, Jimmie and I decided to hire a private physical therapist to come to our home. Miss Maxine Reiser answered our want ad in the *Times Picayune* and agreed to come to our home three days a week.

Jimmie and I found interesting that the first thing she did was teach Jim how to fall and how to put his arms out to protect his head. He had to wear a football helmet to protect his head while he practiced walking on crutches. Three times a week he walked all the way around the block to build up his strength. Maxine was very patient, never pushing too hard nor expecting too much, but always kind with her insistence. However, Jim expected a lot from himself and made himself continue when it was evident he was tired and exhausted. Now it was Jeanne's turn to be happy at seeing her brother learn to walk.

*****

That Christmas morning around five o'clock, we heard, "Mama, Daddy!" as we all tumbled out of bed to see what Santa had brought during the night. Jimmie carried Jim in his arms, and as he pointed to each toy, he let Jim touch them. Jeanne dashed around from toy to toy and squealed when Annette sat in her stroller. Jeanne had a tricycle made from a merry-go-round horse, and Annette had a cuddly little doll. Santa had brought Jim a train mounted on a blue rolling box that would fit under his bed when not in use. Our very best Christmas present was knowing each of our children was happy.

Far away in Clarks, Benita Ann didn't even know it was Christmas although it was being celebrated all around her. But my feeling sad wouldn't help her or help those under my care, so I put those thoughts out my mind.

Jimmie, the children, and I then drove to Thibodaux to

be with the rest of the Peltier family, which had grown even larger. There were now eighteen grandchildren. As all the excitement a big family creates surrounded us, we counted our blessings, not wanting to know what 1959 might bring. We were thankful no one could foresee the future and knew it was best to live one day at a time without any idea of what lay ahead.

Chapter Fourteen

Our First Loss

On April 8, we celebrated Jim's fifth birthday. Even though he walked around for a while on his crutches, he was more comfortable in his stroller. Seeing him blow out his candles, a stranger wouldn't have been able to guess Jim had been ill all those years. He was at ease with the children and their mothers who often visited in the afternoon.

We celebrated Easter in DeRidder that year. Easter has always been my favorite holiday because the Resurrection represents hope, and hope was what I needed most.

On Easter morning Jimmie and I hid the beautifully decorated eggs, hoping our children would have fun finding them. Jim used his stroller to go in search of eggs to fill his basket, but Jeanne didn't rush to find her eggs before Jim could. As they both filled their baskets, we were happy she certainly found her share, but Jeanne seemed to have an understanding far beyond her two-and–one-half years.

*****

April 13 dawned like any other day. But when I picked up Annette to bathe her, she had a blank stare, almost as if a film was over her eyes. She had been very alert over the last few weeks, saying "Hi" to everyone in such an adorable way. When I had seen this same stare in Benita Ann's eyes two years previously, I wasn't sure what it meant nor the seriousness of it all. Now there was no mistake. We had serious troubles.

I called Jimmie at Charity Hospital, interrupting his work once again. Though it wasn't the kind of alarm requiring he meet me at the Mercy Hospital emergency room, I just wanted him to know. Our never hiding anything from each other was very important, and we both knew this new symptom wasn't one offering a good prognosis.

I found Dr. Garcia at the emergency room, but there was nothing he could do for Annette that day, so Annette and I returned home to wait. A few days later, she began having convulsions, the petit mal type seizure in which her arm and her leg would contract rhythmically. The drug Dilantin brought her convulsions under control, and she was admitted into the hospital for observation.

A year and three months had passed since Annette's last operation, but a few days later, a decision was made to remove her shunt. These weeks in the hospital were long, but they were nothing compared to the heartbreak of knowing we had yet another child not aware of the world around her.

No one could explain why the original symptoms of hydrocephalus were no longer with Benita nor with Annette even though some terrible results were left in their wake. Jimmie and I couldn't help wondering if this might also happen to Jim.

May 17, 1959, began normally with Jeanne, Annette, and Jim eating breakfast. Then for no apparent reason, Jim began to convulse. I grabbed him, telling Flora to get Jimmie on the phone and to tell him to call Dr. Garcia and then meet me at Mercy's emergency room. Somewhere I'd heard about using a spoon to prevent the convulsing person from having his tongue fall back, closing his vital airway. As I ran from the house, I quickly picked up a spoon.

The trip to the hospital was interminable. I seemed to get all the red lights as each building and car around me seemed so vivid while I talked to Jim constantly, "Jim, you are O.K.

Don't be frightened. You're going to be all right!"

Having to grab Jim's tongue at moments to hold it forward, I finally arrived at the hospital with him. The doctors stopped the convulsions with sedative injections and then admitted him. Jim lay peacefully for a few minutes, but shortly after we were settled on the fifth floor, his projectile vomiting started with tremendous force. Unable to imagine the sensations Jim felt, I picked him up and held him close again saying, "It's all right. Don't be frightened."

Dr. Garcia immediately gave orders to prepare for emergency surgery as the minutes crept by. With Jim in such distress, all I could do was hold him. Jimmie dashed back to Charity Hospital to complete the procedures he had begun and to make arrangements to get away. By the time Jimmie got back to Jim's hospital room, the nurses were giving Jim the preoperative injections for surgery, so Jimmie had only a few minutes with Jim before he was rolled away.

Our minds were racing, but all Jimmie and I could do was sit down and begin the long wait. As we watched the nurses prepare a bed for a returning surgical patient, Jimmie and I sat in that hospital room while downstairs, our only son, just five years old, once more had to have his shunt revised. Although the procedure sounded so simple, we knew in actuality what complications might occur. We had had no experience as yet with a five year old having this type of surgery. Jim had been the first to undergo brain surgery, so when Benita Ann and Annette had their turns in the operating room, we based our hopes on his past experiences. Veterans as we were, this was one more new road for Mom and Dad, too.

Maybe Jimmie and I wanted our thought processes dulled. We knew Jim's skull bones were now fused together and couldn't separate to allow the fluid to accumulate as when he was a baby. We knew this was the reason for his violent illness. The contrast between waiting for his first surgeries and this surgery was great. We had learned to love this little boy and to know him as a real person. The anxiety we now experienced was more intense than that for his surgeries as a baby. During those other procedures, I thought no surgery could be any worse, but this child had lived with us for five years. We cared for him, watched him develop, loved him and saw him overcome so many hydrocephalic setbacks through these years.

Jim came back to his room at eleven o'clock in the evening as Dr. Garcia again said, "We did what we set out to do!"

Jimmie and I both breathed sighs of relief and said to ourselves, "Thank you, God."

We sat close to Jim's bed to watch his every breath. As we looked at each other across his bed through the night hours, Jim slept peacefully. All his vital signs were normal when the sunlight came through the window in the morning. So we decided Jimmie should go home and bathe and shave in order to begin the new day. After he had his turn at home, I would take mine.

Jimmy hadn't been gone very long when Jim began to have another convulsion. I ran to the nurse's desk for help. The morning shift had just checked in, and the night shift was still there, so people came running from everywhere. So much was happening in such a limited space that someone must have asked me to step out into the hall. I saw them running, pushing a suction machine and an oxygen tank. The central oxygen supply had failed to function, and I had no doubt that caused Jim's convulsions. Looking back and remembering, I still get mad.

I quickly called Jimmie saying, "Jim's in trouble."

Then I just stood in the hall. I'm not sure I was even praying. Anyway, I had prayed so much I felt God was constantly with me, and the Bible says God knows our every need.

Dr. Garcia entered the room, only to walk back out to tell me Jim had died. He made the announcement so simply — his words telling me my world with my little boy was over.

By this time, Jimmie was on his way back, so Dr. Garcia walked up and down the hall in front of the elevators as I talked. I probably said a lot of unnecessary things because my thoughts were so disconnected and flooded my mind. This confusion allowed me a little time to really face what had happened. I guess I cried; I don't know. I wanted Jimmie to get there to share what had happened, but at the same time, I wished for his sake he'd never have to know. But he knew instantly when he got off the elevator and saw me. As Dr. Garcia began to tell him what happened, he just said, "Let's go see Jim."

How different to see Jim after all that fight and spunk I loved the most had left his body. After all the struggle his body had been through in the last twenty-four hours, I was surprised to see his quiet expression. His face was so peaceful in death.

Jim's bed was near a window. Jimmie confided in me later he was stunned when he happened to look outside and saw people going to work. It seemed strange to him that the world was still actively preparing for the day because his day had stopped. Jimmie couldn't even believe the sun had come up.

Just a short time ago, hope and vitality had been in the room. Now there was only silence. The room, the hospital — all felt too small to house such a tragedy. Jimmie and I couldn't help feeling there was something we should do. We wanted to protest to someone that this couldn't be. We felt completely helpless as the nurses and doctors were standing by the door, no one saying much.

When I hear about the death of a first born son, I often wonder whether the parents feel as completely drained, mentally and physically, as the two of us felt that day.

Jimmie and I stood there for a little while, then we finally realized there were things that had to be done – things that were bigger than we – things we couldn't control. This was a time we would have to live through whether we wanted to or not. Our roles had been pre-determined. What would take place now was a ritual set up by mankind long before our time – the ritual of burying our dead.

When we drove back to our house, we found one of Jimmie's

aunts waiting. Someone must have called the Peltier family and asked her to come to be with us until others could arrive from Thibodaux. I found myself looking at her, thinking how hard it must have been for her to come alone and face us, but also thinking how kind she was.

I busied myself polishing Jim's brown shoes and getting out his little suit he wore to church. Each action seemed so deliberate — everything around me so vivid. However, my mind was dull to the realization of what all of this meant to my life.

Jimmie's family put all the necessary arrangements into motion — only asking about the time we wanted for the visitation and the funeral. The duty I couldn't escape and dreaded most was calling my mother to tell her this sad news. Once that was done, I just stood or sat or talked when the occasion dictated. I just did whatever I was told to do.

Like Mary after finding Jesus in the Temple, I filed everything away in my thoughts — thoughts I deliberately waited to have after all the necessary things had been done and I could be alone to sort them out in my own way. The minutes seemed to drag by, but we were actually at our home only a short while before leaving for Thibodaux. I was happy Jeanne was so young and couldn't understand. We decided she and Annette could stay home in Metairie with Flora Kohn, our maid, while we were away.

That very night, only thirty-six hours after our family had enjoyed a normal waking morning, Jimmie and I walked into the funeral home to spend a few private minutes alone with our five-year-old... my child... Jimmie's son... my best friend... lying in a casket.

When I saw Jim, I had to smile. I loved him so much that just seeing him, even like this, made me smile. I was unprepared for this strange reaction, even as it happened. Jim was so absent; his body was there, but his spirit and his soul were gone. The Jim I knew and loved had vanished. There was a tear in his eye that I wiped away. I believe it was symbolic in that it was his last tear, thank God. But not ours.

Many times in the past five years, Jimmie and I met many challenges side by side with our heads held high. That is how we now met Jim's death. Neither of us had a desire to weep and cry or cling to anyone. I really felt this occasion demanded more dignity than that. We wouldn't exhibit in the midst of the public the collapse we inwardly felt.

How did I feel about God at this time? That is hard to describe. I felt I had spent all my minutes each day with Him and had spent formal time praying, but most of all, I had just lived with Him. There were times when I said, "Thank you." And then there were the times I said, "Please help!" But in my life, there wasn't any certain, isolated segment of time set aside for God. He was there all the time. I would have to live through the minutes, the hours, the days knowing He had my child for Himself now.

*****

My first recollection of Thibodaux is of an automobile tour conducted by my new fiancé. As clearly as anything he'd ever told me, I recall his saying during that tour, "Do you see that funeral home? That's where they'll lay you and me out one day." I never dreamed that a part of me would be laid out there only six years later.

The funeral home was jam-packed. Although I had never lived here, I was pleased, if that is possible, to see so many people I knew file through. I hadn't known what such an outpouring of love could be like. People were deeply sorry at our great loss and offered their sympathy to comfort us, but it was our turn to ache. I knew Jimmie and I were the only ones who could truly feel this loss – no one else could.

Before Jimmie and I followed Jim's bier down the long aisle of magnificent St. Joseph Cathedral, I asked at the door if I might place my hand on Jim's coffin and actually help push it to the front altar. I felt like I was truly giving Jim back to God. I had hoped throughout those few years I had him that he would grow up to be a priest. As I slowly approached the altar, I again thought how I would have liked to give Jim to God as an adult. But God must have wanted Jim to be a child with Him in Heaven now instead.

Jim had a white Mass — a Mass of the Angels, the usual requiem for those who die before they reach the age of reason. Reverend Edward Ramagosa, S.J., our cousin whose life had intertwined with ours all of these years and who had sat on the floor to play blocks with Jim just a few months before, came from his parish to offer Jim's Mass of the Angels.

Reverend Ramagosa offered the most beautiful words of consolation to all of us in the congregation about how today Jim was with his Father in Heaven. Each word and thought from the sermon rang true to me as I sat quietly in the pew. At one point, I could hardly hear the homily because Jim's Grandfather Harvey Peltier sobbed so loudly from the pain of his grandchild's death.

I really don't know where I got the endurance which allowed me to sit there quietly while the child I'd given my all to for five years was being eulogized, blessed, and prepared for burial. Surely this extra strength must have come from God. During the Mass, I never thought of myself as a person; I felt I was part of a great happening God was directing. Because He loved me, I wanted to lend the grace, honor, and dignity to Jim's Angel Mass it clearly demanded. All I can say is I lived through Jim's funeral Mass with God. I have no grand statements to describe it. As I placed my hand on Jim's coffin at the end of his funeral Mass, I also took part in removing my baby from the church.

As we drove from the church to the cemetery with a long, long line of cars behind us, words I'd overheard rang in my ears, "Life does go on."

As I stepped out the car, I tripped on the rug. Everyone reached to support me, assuming I was weak and fainting. I wish I had been able to faint; but, alas, I really had tripped. I was very much alive and conscious, more aware than at any other moment in my life.

I'd been asked if it would be easier on us to place Jim's casket into the vault and to close the doors to the vault after we departed. However, I wanted to see everything done and finished completely. I don't know why I was asked to make these decisions. Jimmie's wishes were equally important to me, if not more.

So there in St. Joseph Cemetery, our baby was buried. No one had ever lived five years with more love than the love we gave Jim. We were his legs, his arms, his answer to his every desire. I knew his body from head to toe, even to that mole on his foot over his little toe just like mine. He had received undivided love twenty-four hours a day from two devoted parents. I thanked God for giving him to me and letting me care for him.

At lunch that day, Mr. Peltier said, "Time will heal."

I was infuriated. I felt nothing could ever heal what I felt this day, and, furthermore, I didn't want to be healed. I didn't want time to pass, taking Jim farther away from me, taking from me the warmth of his body. But it is true — much time does soften the rough edges, the sharp hurting the loss of someone you devoted your life to causes.

After Jim's funeral was all over, everyone went to Jimmie's parents' home for a libation. I don't know why French people think a drink is the answer to pain or glory. Maybe it is. I just watched and tried to be part of the group because they were sincerely giving themselves to help Jimmie and me. Each of them felt true sorrow.

I made very few statements about my private thoughts to anybody. However, while Jimmie's family sat around talking, I confided my past dreams for Jim.... How I had wished he would become a priest... How I used to picture him on the altar, celebrating Mass...How I would have seen the scar on the back of his neck as he lifted the Host in reverence. However, it seemed God preferred Jim at the age of five in Heaven with Him.

After telling this story, I was very embarrassed having shared my private feelings. Alone later, I realized I shouldn't have felt embarrassment. These people of French origin are used to expressing their ideas freely and find strength in sharing their emotions — those drinks *did* help. Life *did* go on. Time *did* heal.

Chapter Fifteen

Life Does Go On

After the day of Jim's funeral, I just followed where I was led. Trying to be protective, our family felt Jimmie and I should go fishing in the Louisiana marsh just to get away. This we did. I'm sure Jimmie was only following suggestions and taking the line of least resistance just as I was.

Out on the water surrounded by marsh, Jimmie and I felt suspended in time. The marsh has a beauty all its own. Not a beauty one is immediately aware of; rather, one recognized after many visits. Our earlier trips to the marsh had been short pleasure trips, but after the overpowering loss of our child, we found a solitude there that provided needed therapy and a sense of timelessness. Those few quiet days of watching the calm sun rise and set offered Jimmie and me a special comfort before we had to pick up the pieces and meet life ahead again. We knew we would meet the challenge, but it was good to know there was always a quiet retreat waiting for us if needed.

When we tied up the boat and looked back at the quietness such an escape had given us, we longed to run away from reality a little longer, but our responsibilities were once again taking shape in our thoughts. We forced ourselves to turn around and look ahead.

Running away, even to go fishing, can only last so long;

our bodies had to return home, and our minds had to return to think of others. Back home waiting for us we had Jeanne, that beautiful little brunette with curly hair, and Annette, who needed to be handled with hands of love. Jim had been a minute-by-minute part of Jeanne's life, but even at three years of age, Jeanne was visibly affected by his death. With effort, this could be overcome. After having a house full with four babies, we were suddenly down to two. Jim was in Heaven, and Benita Ann in Clarks. Nothing remains static.

*****

Jimmie and I worked conscientiously at keeping busy. The hours I had filled with Jim, I was now filling with Jeanne and Annette. I loved Jimmie and the girls; I cooked, smiled and the time seemed to pass. In addition, we were making the move to Thibodaux in just three weeks. We'd be back home. Because it was Jimmie's home, it became my home, too.

Jimmie and I were still trying to abstain sexually. We just couldn't have another baby; so now we only needed one baby bed. We packed those dear pieces of furniture that had been Jim's. The movers were so efficient they'd have even packed dirty pots and moved them if they were left unattended for a minute.

Jeanne, our maid Flora, and I went to Thibodaux several times to clean the house we were moving into. It was good we were leaving the Camphor Street home where Jim had been the center of attention every minute. It would be good to have a different environment for Jeanne. All her cousins would be in Thibodaux for her to learn to know and to love.

One cousin Jimmie's age said, "Just wait until you get Jeanne to Thibodaux. She'll give up her corrective shoes and get more than one baby doll to carry around."

Before this move, our family life had been limited to just a mother, a father and children. In Thibodaux, we'd associate daily with grandparents, aunts, uncles, and cousins. Our children would be exposed to other people's ways of doing things. Until now, Jimmie and I had easily directed our children's actions. We controlled the food they ate, carefully limiting sweets. We chose their clothes. Now they would observe their peers and observe other households in action.

That cousin was correct. Jeanne would see the little black patent sandals and prefer them to corrective oxfords. She would discover other kinds of dolls, and the one little doll she had lavished such love on would take a back seat.

*****

Jimmie and I discovered a curious difference in our separate reactions to Jim's death. I wanted to think about Jim as frequently as I could. Jimmie could only help himself by not thinking of him. Over a year passed before Jimmie would even bring himself to look at home movies again.

I missed Jim in so many ways. I'd carried Jim in my arms for five years. I'd carried him all around the house, down cafeteria lines, down store aisles. I missed holding him and the warmth of his body. I missed the times I just kissed his cheek or forehead. I missed touching him. I'd held him close so he wouldn't feel alone or frightened.

I thought of Jim in Heaven. I tried to imagine what Heaven must be like from what I'd read in the Bible. Jesus said, "In my Father's house, there are many mansions. I go to prepare a place for you," but I couldn't believe a little boy would be very happy in a mansion. I'd led Jim to believe I'd always be there to take care of him. Now I wondered who was there and what his life would be like. No amount of yearning for this knowledge could reveal all this to me.

I love God and believe Jim to be happy with Him. I wanted Jim to have the happiness he must have missed on earth, I thought of him as if he sat in a big comfortable chair – softness all around him. I wanted him to sink into the softness and comfort and to enjoy being with God.

I didn't want to deprive Jim of any happiness by my grieving. If my sorrow could be seen by Jim, it might make him feel sad. I didn't want him to have any heartaches, just happiness. So consciously, I tried not to weep just in case my pain would hurt him.

Deep inside, I always felt a little guilty I'd left one thing undone in Jim's life — his receiving the Sacrament of Confirmation. A child is usually confirmed around the age of ten after his first communion and confession. I thought I was rearing Jim to manhood; therefore, I didn't have him confirmed early. Many Roman Catholics believe the sacraments contribute to a person's degree of happiness in Heaven. I wanted the highest degree of happiness for Jim in Heaven. Our priest assured me Jim was as totally happy in Heaven as the saintliest saint.

I wrote notes to people who'd been kind enough to show sympathy with their soothing words and their flowers for Jim's death. I even wrote to the people who just came to the funeral home and signed their names to the visitor's book because their being there was a tribute to our son. Each note was written with sincerity. I wrote them with as much meaning as I could possibly draw from within the depths of myself. I performed this task to the very best of my ability, but how can a person use ordinary words formed from the twenty-six letters of the alphabet to say what is felt for the love poured out over the death of a treasured child? How could I say thank you adequately?

I was surprised at the number of beautiful letters we received. The letter dearest to me came from Miss Maxine Reiser, the physical therapist who'd come to our home regularly to teach Jim to walk. She spoke of a discouraging time in her life, a turning point in her life. She needed to decide whether she should continue in physical therapy.

She wrote, "I was tempted to follow the easy direction and call it all off, but after seeing such push and drive, after seeing the demands a young boy had made on his body and energies, I decided that I, too, would be capable of making demands on myself. Jim could have said no because he knew the loving situation he was in and that no one would have *made* him continue. But day after day, I saw him drive himself, no matter how tired or how many times he fell. Therefore, I decided I could also meet the challenge. If it is any consolation, please know your young son has helped shape my life to make a decision that will cause me to be a finer person."

I couldn't help wondering how many of us in a lifetime would affect another life and make another person better for having known us. What an influence our young son had been!

Chapter Sixteen

Thibodaux, Louisiana

$\mathcal{J}$immie, our children, and I moved to Thibodaux, finally going to a place where a lot of people loved us simply because we were family. Because the Louisiana French country is a place always ready to welcome someone new, friends of our family accepted us as we were. People there had all heard about our troubles and welcomed us with open arms. I felt good to be a part of an old farming community – and a part of a grand, large family.

Jimmie liked moving into his new office, one constructed and designed using a novel idea for 1959. Because the roof was poured on the ground and then lifted, the building was a first for Thibodaux. This lift-slab roof drew crowds of sidewalk superintendents as it was successfully completed and raised into place.

At this time, there were no oral surgeons in South Louisiana, so Jimmie's first case in private practice was in Lake Charles, Louisiana, two hundred miles away. Jimmie flew there to remove an imbedded part of a broken hypodermic needle from a man's throat. This first case was very difficult, but meeting this challenge gave Jimmie the good feeling he needed and wanted. This case launched his surgical practice, and we began our new life with joy.

Jimmie and I were still young, just twenty-eight years old.

My goodness, so much had happened in twenty-eight years! We still counted days of sexual abstinence, hoping to bring no more children into this world. But because of Jim's death, my ovulation time had been thrown off completely. My God, I was pregnant again! Surely, our heartaches were all behind us. A healthy child must be on the way. A new home, a new life, and a new baby arriving in less than a year!

Annette developed a terrible diaper rash, one that seemed to baffle everybody. We went to several dermatologists and tried to come to grips with an unusually difficult case. Every imaginable medication applied locally and administered orally was tried. Finally, doctors suggested she be left without a diaper so fresh air could reach her affected area. This meant Annette needed someone to sit by her every minute. If the rash itched, she had to be prevented from scratching.

After several days, we hired someone to sit with Annette at least five hours each afternoon so we could have a break. She did get better, but we were again hearing from the doctors that she should be placed in a home for exceptional children. Clarks was a wonderful place. Benita Ann was receiving excellent care there.

Again I didn't listen to those suggestions — I just ignored their advice. I felt Annette was too young, and we certainly had enough time to care for her. In fact, I had been thinking that perhaps we should bring Benita Ann back home since Jim was gone and we now had more time to care for her.

Several of our Louisiana friends were going to a dental meeting in New York. Jimmie and I wanted to go very much; we needed a break. We tried to remember whether or not I had done anything unusual during my other pregnancies which might have caused our babies to have hydrocephalus. I had read that during some airplane flights, a possible lack of oxygen at high altitudes might cause changes for an expectant mother and harm the baby. During my other pregnancies, I had flown to Boston several times. But Jeanne had been born healthy, so that disproved this theory. Surely, our babies being sick had nothing to do with my flying.

I did, however, convince Jimmie we should take the train to New York instead because of the remote possibility that air travel had some relationship to hydrocephalus. I'd have to return home on the train alone while Jimmie flew home because he had surgery scheduled. Morning nausea is one thing, but vomiting on a moving train is terrible. However, I'd have done anything to ensure our having a healthy baby.

I must have enjoyed the trip — the gourmet restaurants, the stores, the general excitement of being in New York — but I had many worries in the back of my mind, including my loneliness for Jim and my concern about my pregnancy. I told myself everyone had to be somewhere to pass the time away, and certainly New York with Jimmie would be a grand way to pass that time. I'd always been thankful we could afford to take nice trips, live comfortably, and have the special amenities that enriched our lives. Those extras helped sustain our positive attitudes in the face of so much discouragement and despair.

*****

Books offered the best escape from remembering and thinking, so the first place I visited in Thibodaux had been the parish library. Sometimes reading about generations of other families with all their trials and tribulations helped me see our life as a total happening rather than just isolated, pointed heartaches that seemed to occupy such endless hours and days. Stories in those books reminded me of all the traumas others throughout all time have had to endure and will always continue to endure. After reading these novels, I didn't feel so much like a separate individual going through these times alone. I felt like a part of a universe that has ups and downs. Books helped me see life in a wider scope.

Our home in Thibodaux offered a change from anything we'd previously known. There were many couples our own age, and Jimmie had grown up with most of them. I played bridge each time I was invited to do so. We joined all the clubs we were invited to join. One civic club even invited me to become a member before we had left New Orleans.

I tried to be aware of the world around me. I didn't want to get caught up in my daily routine and miss everything going on just because my life seemed abnormal compared to that of my friends. I worked at getting others to talk. From my reading, I knew others welcomed the opportunity to talk, especially about themselves. I tried desperately never to complain. If anyone inquired about my family, I always replied, "Better. Things are better now."

I was always amazed at how people complained about "My headache" or "My cold" or that "My child is teething" or "My child has colic." To them, these minor annoyances were as serious a problem as they could conceive at the moment.

It was interesting people knowing my circumstances never seemed to think, "I have a cold, but she just lost a child and has two more she will probably lose. A cold is not as overpoweringly important as her discomfort."

In all the years of our troubles, very few people seemed to think that deeply. Knowing surgery was scheduled the next day for my baby, they would visit me in the hospital and spend the whole time talking about the worst thing that had ever happened to them, like a dent in a fender.

I would try to direct all my attention to truly listening to their problems — really listening with concern — as I wished someone would listen to me or Jimmie. It became a game to me. I learned not to blame them at all. I didn't even feel agitated with them.

I frequently made an effort to be at certain places that weren't always exciting simply to make friends and nurture friendships. I played bridge and belonged to my civic clubs with that as my main objective. I wanted to learn. I wanted to have new experiences each day so I could offer new conversation and new ideas to my husband and children. Without Jim, I had more time. I decided that rather than feeling sorry for myself, I'd participate in everything offered me in the community, even to the point of urging myself on when I didn't want to go.

My mind wandered daily to my longing for Jim. The blankness, *no* contact, *no* signs from Heaven were ever felt. The helplessness of it all continued to engulf me. My goodness, I had prayed and felt close to God. It all felt very one-sided— one-sided on my side. I did all the talking and imagining, but I never really ever heard anything from God.

I certainly didn't expect Him to talk to me. I wasn't worthy to even think such a thought, but I felt surely there must be some way I could be sure He was there — not from the Bible and what others before me had written and said, but some way all my own. Surely, there must be a sign for me.

No such encouragement came, but with the faith God had given me, there must have been some courage coming from Him. I still prayed; I still believed. What else could I do? I was pregnant again. Perhaps that would be the sign. Maybe God would give me a healthy baby. Jimmie and I were only twenty-eight years old then. It would be like starting over in a way. We'd have Jeanne and the new baby. We could make an attempt at a new life. Maybe that was what God had in mind.

Now I had time to humor myself and think in spite of nausea and vomiting being my constant companions. Cooking and taking care of Jeanne and Annette left me little extra time. Jimmie began to play golf often, I suppose to prevent his having time to think.

I found myself having morbid thoughts. I knew no one else was aware of them, but I had to work hard to prevent those thoughts from returning over and over. Whenever I drove by the big Peltier tomb in the cemetery, I'd think of the vacuum in there – the lack of air, the feeling of being closed in, and what a prisoner of war would feel in isolation with the hot sun baking down on a concrete chamber. I began taking other streets to reach my destination so I wouldn't have to pass by that big tomb with the black door.

After the first four months of my pregnancy were finally over, I never had those thoughts again, even if I drove by the tomb. Months later, I couldn't imagine my ever having had such morbid thoughts. That must have been a very low time for me. I would never have volunteered this information because I knew it wasn't healthy to live with this kind of thinking, so no one realized how despondent I was.

Christmas 1959 was to be the first Jimmie and I celebrated in Thibodaux. My parents were going to Kosciusko, Mississippi, to be with my mother's relatives. Our plans were to have Christmas in our own home and then go over to the Peltier family for Christmas dinner. So much is said and written about the joy at Christmas time that some people are unhappy because they believe they are supposed to be exuberant and aren't.

For very different reasons, this was a very sad Christmas for me. My mother called and said that each year during all the time she had been a teacher, she had read *The Littlest Angel* to her class. After losing Jim, she could never read that story again.

This was about the time the Christmas carol *The Little Drummer Boy* began to sweep the country. I could not listen to it because it brought thoughts of Jim back so vividly.

As well as I knew every detail of Jim's countenance, I felt his image slipping away from me. I hated for time to pass because time drew Jim farther away from me. Why is it a human mind can't remember and be able to picture exactly what a person looks like when that person is out of sight? Is this what people mean when they say time heals?

Chapter Seventeen

Expecting Our Fifth Child

*O*ne of Jimmie's first cousins was to be ordained a priest in Rome in January 1960. Jimmie, two relatives and a friend decided to attend the ordination and flew there in one of the first commercial jets to cross the Atlantic. That only six hours after leaving New York Jimmie could step down on European soil seemed fantastic. I was happy there was such a happy diversion for Jimmie. This would give him a change of pace. Then, too, I hoped all the extra prayers offered in a hallowed spot like Rome would somehow be effective. I had been told that a child at his first communion receives what he asks for in prayer, so a newly-ordained priest's prayers might be especially powerful. In these restless days, I accepted anything that might do some good.

The days Jimmie were gone were very lonely. I couldn't go home to visit my parents because I certainly couldn't take Annette, and she couldn't be left behind. During this time, I began practicing playing the piano again, filling some time playing old pieces of music. I deliberately tried to keep busy, going from cooking to cleaning and then to reading.

I had to help myself! I had no such thing as a best friend There were many I called friends, but there was no particular one in whom I could confide. That was a luxury I knew I couldn't afford because I wouldn't want anyone to have to really share my heartaches. I felt all our friends watched us from afar and felt sorry we had such troubles. I couldn't and wouldn't pull them any closer into my web of pain. And they kept their safe distance.

Despite my apprehension, my being pregnant was a joy. To have a baby growing inside of me gave me an especially good feeling, a feeling of purpose — a feeling of being involved in a miracle — a feeling of doing something unusual all by myself.

I felt very close to God knowing He had one of my children. I continually reminded myself that all my children were God's children and that He had only loaned them to me for a time on earth, even if they felt like mine alone. I reminded myself that God is Love and that He loved my children more than I ever could, but I knew I loved them as much as was humanly possible. My mind battled many thoughts while I waited for Jimmie to return from Rome. When he was near me, his presence prevented me from thinking thoughts that might be better left alone.

Jimmie did return safely; and yes, he'd prayed ever so hard at all the right places in Rome. We seemed again to be begging and waiting. Jimmie had almost been granted an audience with Pope John XXIII. He'd even reached the Pope's antechamber and heard his voice. But the Pope was anxious to begin a retreat, so the audience was denied. Jimmie's trip had been wonderful; however, having him home again was also wonderful.

With our having a healthy baby, a three-year-old girl, and the arrival of our new baby, we'd almost be starting over again with a new family and a different vision for the future. I couldn't allow myself to think God had other plans.

After seven years of marriage, life had changed completely for me and Jimmie. We didn't have to struggle with our daily anxieties about hydrocephalus with Jim; Benita Ann was settled at Clarks; and four-year-old Annette lay in her bed all day like an infant. Care for Annette consisted of keeping her clean and well fed. Jeanne was a beautiful, healthy three-year-old, curly headed little girl. And now I awaited our fifth baby.

I was able to concentrate on keeping house, dressing each child in pretty clothes, and enjoying time. No longer was I driven to snatch a few minutes here and there to read or just broil a veal chop quickly for meals. I now had time, glorious time, to fill as I saw fit. After so much tension, setting such a relaxed pace was difficult. Many afternoons, I could bathe, redress myself and put a fresh dress and spotless white shoes on Jeanne to visit my sister-in-law. After having lived a life of rushing every minute with hydrocephalus night and day, my new life tantalized me.

Living in the Deep South with a yard of our own, Jimmie discovered a new hobby — growing camellias — and became deeply involved in all phases. I was happy he found pleasure reading about the subject and working with the plants. The tender, loving care he provided produced quality blooms we could all appreciate. He even won some competitive camellia shows.

One of our new friends was Father Jerome Ropollo, the pastor of a small parish near Thibodaux. We'd met him at a small, casual supper party we attended. Occasionally we'd invite him to dinner at our home. Naturally, our conversations drifted to our anxiety about the health of our coming baby. The three of us spent many hours discussing religion. Nearly everywhere we went in the late fifties, Catholicism was discussed. Almost all our friends were true, practicing Catholics, all having large families and keeping their promise not to practice artificial birth control. This wasn't easy for any of these couples because the subject came up frequently.

Father Ropollo was a jovial, happy priest with the capacity to be comfortable in a man's world as well as in a female's. He assured us our new baby would be normal and healthy. Why not? He'd seen all the good God gives this world. He knew we were faithful Catholics, and he really felt we wouldn't encounter the same heartaches again.

Jimmie kept saying to him, "Please help me if this baby is sick. I'm going to need help."

I felt I just blundered on toward the big happening in a confused sort of way. I couldn't prepare myself for the good or the bad. I could only place myself in God's hands, try to pray, and try to mean, "Thy will be done."

While waiting, there was no need to curtail our activities. We had guests over for dinner, hosted cocktail parties, and attended parties in town. Jimmie had a drive to take advantage of everything we were offered. If I found myself reticent about participating, I'd remind myself of his drive. He never allowed me to sit still and think – he wanted us to be where the action was. Loving him as I did, I wanted to keep up and take part.

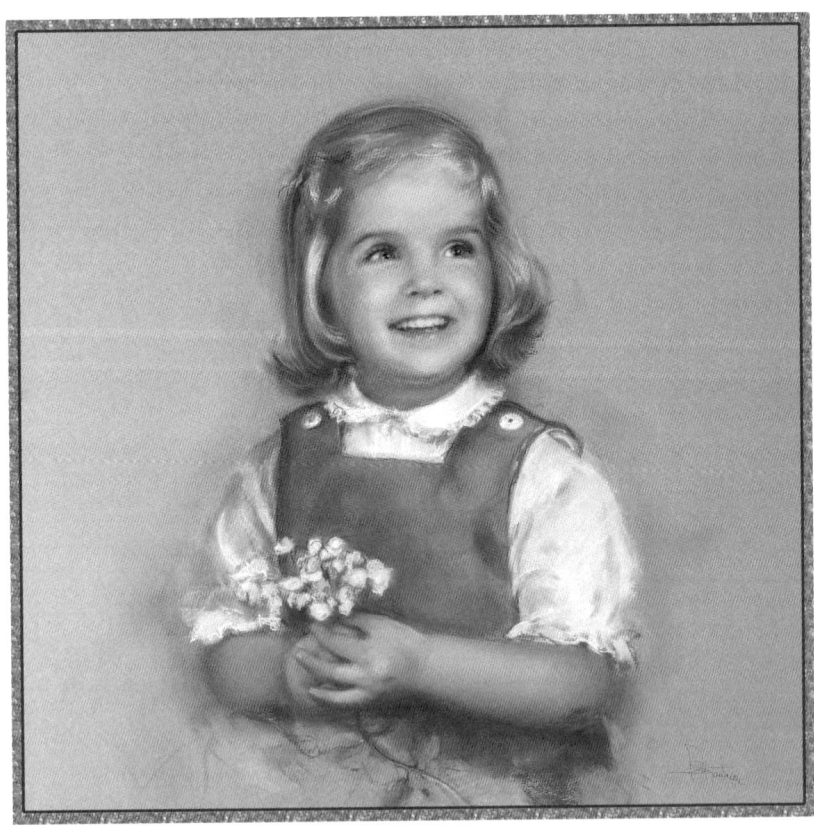

Adrienne Elizabeth Peltier

*****

When my labor pains started, we took only a few minutes to reach St. Joseph Hospital. Because no rooms were available, my labor and a few hours following delivery were spent in a closet once used for mops, brooms and buckets. That inconvenience went practically unnoticed by us – we just wanted to know what our baby's fontanel would feel like after her birth.

I wasn't able to touch her head until I returned from the delivery room. Although the doctors and Jimmie told me all was well, with my first touch, I knew instantly it wasn't. It wasn't a bulging soft spot, but neither was it a sunken one. I asked immediately that a "no visitors" sign be put on my door. I didn't want to see anyone. I just wanted to disappear and not have to face what was obviously in store. We kept telling ourselves that the possibility of the trauma of being born had caused this temporary difference in her fontanel, but we all knew better. The hours that followed were sheer torment. Jimmie spent time with me in my hospital room, but he had to be alone to face our new problem himself.

My mother had come to get Jeanne when I had entered the hospital, so only Annette was at home, and I had someone trustworthy to take care of her.

Adrienne Elizabeth Peltier, born March 4, 1960, was beautiful! She had a perfectly formed body, a lovely shaped head with blonde hair, and her skin wasn't blemished nor red as so many babies' skin is at birth. Her cry was strong and healthy as was her heartbeat. Everything was perfect, except for the minute opening that should be draining her head. I prayed so hard for a miracle and that the obstruction would open. There are so many normal babies born, surely one more normal baby wouldn't bother anybody.

If God would permit Adrienne to be well, I would be happy to sink into the world, and no one would ever notice us. I even wished I'd been able to hide us away from God so He wouldn't do this to our baby.

A priest would admonish me, "God doesn't do this. He permits it to happen."

To me, that was the same. Not only does God permit, He could change the situation and cure her if He wished, which is what I prayed for in my despair. I felt as if I'd had three trial runs with children with hydrocephalus. It was as if I'd practiced and was finally honed to care for a fourth child facing the same horrors. If I'd missed any heartaches on the first three runs, I'd now have a mature mind, a sufferable mind to be hurt more than ever because now I knew too much.

In a small town, this kind of news sweeps through the community with the speed of lightning. I wanted to tell my three bridge partners myself because having these problems was hard for others to talk about to me.

When my friends arrived, we chatted for a while as I was trying to get my courage up to say, "Adrienne has hydrocephalus." I'd planned to be as calm as I'd always made myself be when speaking of this illness.

However, as soon as I got the words out, I burst out crying and was very embarrassed about my losing control. I certainly hadn't meant to cause a scene, but my crying made the situation more human. I think my three friends saw me in a more normal light instead of my trying to appear to be brave all of the time. Even though I let others hear the news about Adrienne through the grapevine, I strongly felt that to be a true friend, I had to tell my close group in my own way.

In our small town hospital, a new mother who recovers from delivery well goes home the following day, but I stayed an extra two days. I was trying to get myself together before I went home to begin again.

Jimmie used those two nights to talk into the wee hours of the morning with Father Ropollo to try to get some understanding and some direction for his thinking. Oh, he had shaken his fist at Heaven on a few occasions — something I considered normal, but now there was a completely different expression on his face.

Right there in the hospital room a few hours after Adrienne's birth, Jimmie and I made the decision to practice artificial means of birth control. During our eight years of marriage, we had never for one second dreamed of taking this course; but after our having four children out of five born with hydrocephalus, we felt we had no other choice. We could no longer think of ourselves; we had to stop bringing any more children into the world to suffer. We felt beaten down by everything. Here we were, parents who loved children, wanted children, and, unmistakably, should have no more.

After reaching that decision, Jimmie and I knew we'd no longer be able to receive Holy Communion when we attended Mass because we'd now be living in a state of mortal sin. I realized the Holy Communion I had received in the hospital that morning would be my last. I had always found joy and comfort from receiving God's body. This would no longer be available to me — just when I felt I needed that sacrament the most.

All seemed so unfair. Jimmie and I had wanted a large family. If we could have had healthy children, we wouldn't need to use artificial birth control. It is terrible to have to decide coldly and with calculation to commit a sin, but I certainly didn't feel I would be sinning. Now when offering my joys, works and sufferings to God each morning, I'd have another suffering to add to the list. Before this, I at least believed my life was right with God, but now I was out of step with that private part of my life that sustained me. I wished I could have stood face to face with God to defend myself.

As I watched Jimmie, I knew this was the hardest decision he'd ever made. He'd been a devout Catholic all of his life. To abandon the beliefs of a lifetime was devastating. We felt so hurt by God. We'd always been taught He was our loving Father. He even knew the number of hairs we had on our heads. He loved us more than our earthly fathers. However, what He kept allowing to happen didn't seem to indicate He loved us very much. I never could have treated children I loved that way. Our child having been born healthy would have affected no one's life other than ours. It would only have given joy.

My thoughts began to wander along many different lines. Maybe God did love us. If our children had to be ill, maybe He chose us very carefully, knowing we would make their years on earth as happy as possible. Maybe allowing us such intense suffering would assure our worthiness to enter Heaven. In reality, we knew we had been pushed too far for the stamina we had as human beings. Jimmie and I had reached the breaking point.

Two days after Adrienne's birth, Jeanne had told my mother, "We have waited all this time for the baby, and I have to go home to see if I can help take care of her."

My mother, being very kind and sensitive to children, did the right thing and brought Jeanne home. Jeanne gave us reason to smile and be brave. Seeing our little three-and-a-half year old, curly-headed brunette playing and giggling made us realize the world hadn't actually ended. We had her to rear and love. I was happy she knew she should come home.

For a few days, Jimmie didn't spend as much time with me as usual. I knew it was because he had to think things through. I had to give him the time he needed.

Adrienne looked like any other beautiful baby bundled in a baby blanket. When Jimmie came to the emergency room exit to take me home, Sister Ucarie, the nun in charge of the nursery, walked behind my wheelchair carrying Adrienne. She took great pride in being part of the happy departure from the hospital for new mothers and their babies. People peeked into the blanket and commented on how pretty our baby was. There were big smiles on everyone's face. I looked straight ahead and thought, *If you only knew!*

I loved feeding Adrienne, changing her diapers, and just being home with her and listening to her breathe. I liked standing by and watching her little hands and arms stretch out and contract while she slept or seeing her ball her fist up and rub her eyes. She had a healthy cry, but I was so over-anxious that she had little occasion to exercise her lungs. The moments

I held her were precious. I wanted to hold her close and will a different future for her.

People left us alone, baffled and confused about what to say or do for us. All the beautiful words of faith had been said the other three times, words about miracles and God's goodness. I believe even the most devout, optimistic people by now had no bright words about help and hope.

This time I didn't call any nuns or priests, expecting positive results when they stormed Heaven with prayer. If they were interested, they'd hear our news, and they could pray. Prayers weren't answered the way we wanted them to be. I was a little disgruntled with all the saints, in particular, St. Anne de Beaupre — all those intercessions that seemingly went unanswered.

I had delivered on all my promises even though the answer I wanted had never come. Fifty dollars to this church, forty dollars to that mission, a rosary every day, so many short prayers to Jesus, Mary and Joseph. My struggle to know the Blessed Mother seemed hopeless. I felt they'd all turned their backs on us. I even went to Confession to say I was sorry for having such uncharitable thoughts about the saints.

The Catholic Church taught me to pray to saints, asking them to intercede with God for special requests, so my mind naturally wandered to Jim in Heaven. He was a saint; maybe I should pray to him for help, but somehow I hated to ask him. All the saints I had troubled with my prayers either didn't hear or didn't ask God because none of what I'd begged for had ever materialized. I wouldn't ask Jim. I didn't want to do anything to give me grounds for doubting Jim's ability to ask God. I couldn't leave myself vulnerable to being turned down by him.

Continuously I heard, "Prayers are always answered, not maybe in the way we want them to be, but God hears our prayers."

I felt I had enough experience at twenty-nine to know as a fact my prayers weren't answered as I wished. Whether

God hears all prayers and guides us, I'd just have to wait and see.

I watched Jimmie trying to be courageous. When he didn't know I was near, I watched him pick Adrienne up ever so gently. There was a combination of love and tragedy in every line on his face.

For the first time in my life, I couldn't think happy thoughts or make light conversation. In the past, I could at least work at diverting our thoughts with interest in a fine bottle of wine or a special meal, but now nothing held any interest for me.

Chapter Eighteen

Back To Mercy Hospital

*D*r. Garcia saw no need to examine Adrienne before his admitting her into the hospital. After her body had grown a little and her anatomy developed somewhat, he said we could then come with her to Mercy Hospital prepared for surgery.

Just twenty days after her birth and her little body not seeming much longer, Adrienne was admitted into the hospital.

Here we were again. Back in the hospital on the same fifth floor. Father Ropollo had driven with us to admit Adrienne and stayed for a time. But Jimmie and I found ourselves once again looking into each other's eyes across our child's hospital bed.

I felt so close to Jimmie. We had taken every step of these illnesses together, and he had never shirked a minute of his responsibility. Some men would have looked for excuses to run, but not Jimmie. This time, I felt we were in a deep, dark, bottomless pool — in water we knew too much about — in water we wished we didn't know about.

Had this been our first tragic experience, we could have looked across that hospital bed with our child between us with more hope. But we knew only too well we were again in an impossible situation. We didn't hide this from each other; but being optimistic people, we managed a small bit of hope for our beautiful baby. Even now, Adrienne seemed so bright and alert, her eyes constantly observing all around her. With all the odds against us and in spite of the past, there seemed to be a silent commitment between us that we were ready to fight again for our baby's life and for her happiness. We each stood as the door to the hospital room slowly opened to once again admit Dr. Garcia. It was as if we had shed our past and had taken up this new cross, a cross we'd carry with perseverance and dignity.

After failing to achieve significant success with the Torkildson operation on our other children, Dr. Garcia now had other ideas. Instead of placing the tubing in the back of Adrienne's neck to connect to the reservoir, he now felt a longer tubing from her head to her abdomen would provide the best drainage. With the tubing in this position, Adrienne could be allowed to grow until an increase in her body length indicated the tube needed to be lengthened. Such a procedure would easily be accomplished by splicing the tubing in the middle. In 1960, this operation was thought to have a better percentage of success.

I don't know who made the decision, but when around-the-clock nurses were ordered because they were necessary for this serious surgery, I was told I was needed at home with Jimmie and Jeanne. Our lives were in upheaval, so my presence at home would help us feel more normal for a time.

After being advised to follow this plan, I could understand the thinking. Adrienne was so young. She didn't know me, and this surgery required nurses anyway. Although it wasn't really necessary, I'd always be with her at night. There would be plenty of time in her life after she did know me when I wouldn't be able to leave Adrienne. I painfully realized now I should think of Jeanne and Jimmie's happiness and must prepare myself for whatever the future would hold.

By now Jeanne was in nursery school. Each morning after she left for school, I'd drive the sixty-five miles to New Orleans, visit Adrienne, and then drive back in time to be home when Jeanne came home from school in the afternoon.

We were fortunate Jeanne was a happy child and very trusting of us. She loved to be with children her own age, so she loved school. With three cousins her own age plus plenty of friends, she always had someone with whom she could play. Jimmie and I were with her every morning and night to give her fatherly and motherly attention. We never let Jeanne see us cry or hear our in-depth conversations about our new tragedy. We explained Adrienne was sick and needed to be in New Orleans for a little operation. She'd be well and would come home soon. I knew Jeanne wasn't discouraged nor did she understand to any great extent.

Those daily trips back and forth to New Orleans gave me more time alone to live with my thoughts. Growing in drainage ditches along the highway were millions of beautiful lavender hyacinths. Each time I passed this gorgeous expanse of flowers in all of their perfection, I had ugly thoughts about the inequities of nature, about that small imperfection in each of my four children.

Many ventriculo-peritoneal shunts worked on the very first try. Babies would be admitted to the hospital, have this surgery, stay to have the stitches removed, and go home. But we never experienced a shunt working on the first insertion with any of our children.

On April 18, 1960, almost a month after her first surgery, Adrienne had to again go through those swinging doors to have her shunt revised. Once her incision had been reopened, the surgeons had to replace her ventricular catheter with a new one. We had to go through yet another eight-hour wait. Jimmie found that five milligrams of Valium enabled him to doze while we kept our vigil, and he always claimed it helped to pass the time.

Jimmie and I made our usual update calls to our family. I felt so sorry for them because no one knew what to do or say, and neither did we. But I always knew my mother was there, thinking of us each minute. I really suffered for the heartaches she experienced and believe they were even greater than ours because she was worried about us as well as our child.

Now we'd have another member of our family with hydrocephalus to take home before long, the pediatricians and doctors urged us to take Annette to Clarks with Benita Ann. So much had happened to us that I thought this move could be made without thinking or feeling. But there's no way one can pick up a three year old baby and move her away from her bed and home without dying a little inside.

Our innocent little girl had struggled through life to eighteen months of age. After her bout with meningitis, she knew and was aware of nothing. She became a total care patient. If we hadn't had another sick child, Annette could have remained with us, but through no one's fault, she had a little sister born with her same deforming, debilitating condition.

All the adult minds felt Annette could have better care in a special home. I don't know how adult I felt with this, but the decision was made, and it was up to me to be brave and face this next step.

We chose a Sunday when Adrienne was having a good day to drive Annette to north Louisiana to be admitted to St. Mary's home in Clarks. Once more, I found myself having to accept a situation whether I liked it or not. To be fair to Jeanne and Adrienne, Annette would have to be placed with the nuns, but that didn't make it an easy duty to perform. I knew I'd visit her often, but I knew she'd never share our home again. Someone else would hear her cries and give her food and bodily care.

With all those tormenting thoughts, we drove to Clarks, did our part and came back in a single day. A day seems to be made up of many endless hours when an unpleasant task has to be accomplished.

Time passed in spite of our misery. Jimmie's practice had grown. He could lose himself for hours at his office. In addition to my daily duties, eating, watching TV, and sleeping helped fill the days.

I drove daily to New Orleans to visit Adrienne, still

sandwiching my trips between school departure and return for Jeanne. On some days, I'd go back with Jimmie after work, and we'd take Jeanne. The nuns often allowed Jeanne to come up to the fifth floor to see her sister when no one was looking. In fact, I believe those were the doctor's orders.

Adrienne was like a picture of health at each stage of her development. The hydrocephalus had surely not affected her appetite. We could see the magnetism she was developing in spite of her encumbrances. Her cooing sounds were like strains of beautiful music in that hospital room. Her eyes were amazingly alert. When she began to look right at us and smile while she kicked her feet and waved her arms, we felt an angel was smiling at us. I was thrilled when Adrienne singled me out for one of her favors. Even though she saw me for only a few hours every day, she seemed to know what role I played in her life because she actually gave me special attention.

With private duty nurses twenty-four hours a day, Adrienne received much more attention than the other babies. She made her promenade in a wheelchair on a pillow instead of in a stroller. Literally, she was the darling of the hospital. I was a little jealous because the nurses were taking care of her and not I. Adrienne was a beautiful sight in her little hospital gown, and, even at this early age, she directed what went on around her.

Adrienne's shunt refused to drain perfectly, so the days and weeks stretched into months. Jimmie and I waited. Time seemed so long! Some of our most anxious hours were spent seeing her head getting larger and nothing being done to stop the growth. Jimmie and I always felt she would get well, and we didn't like seeing her head circumference increase.

Then on May 13, 1960, a little more than two months and a few days after Adrienne's birth, Dr. Garcia decided to try the newest form of surgery, the ventriculo-cardiac shunt. This procedure had been introduced in 1956 by Dr. Eugene B. Spitz, a neurosurgeon at the Children's Hospital in Philadelphia.

The fluid from Adrienne's head would drain into one of

the chambers of her heart by his inserting a permanent Holter valve tubing between her brain and her jugular vein. There was no way for the fluid to re-enter her brain after it had drained because the valve didn't allow for any back-up. The fluid could only go in one direction — out.

There seemed to be no end to what would be done next to treat hydrocephalus. Now Adrienne's heart would be involved as well as her brain. Jimmie and I knew, of course, that we had to allow whatever was presented to us as the solution for Adrienne's problem. Guilty feelings always overcame me as we signed papers giving permission to perform one surgery after another. Our baby was so helpless and defenseless, and our options were so limited.

This surgical procedure lasted longer than ever. After ten hours that seemed to be endless, Dr. Garcia walked in as unperturbed as ever and said, "We did what we had set out to do."

We were all limp after this procedure, but what else could we do but hold our heads high and smile with hope? I had ceased begging God. If He wanted to help, my baby needed help. Now I just existed and waited.

This new shunt seemed to be working well. There were two long months of daily visits to Mercy Hospital before Adrienne was finally discharged. What a happy day July 11 was when we could remove Adrienne's little white hospital gown, put on a brightly colored dress, and all return to Thibodaux.

Our family size was constantly changing. It went from one, two, three, four, then back to three with Benita Ann at Clarks, then back to two without Benita Ann and Jim, and then to one when Annette moved to Clarks and Jeanne was with us alone. Now we were back to two with Adrienne and Jeanne. I still can scarcely believe it all happened.

What a different lifestyle we began! Jeanne, almost four, was the ideal little girl, very much a little girl, very loving, an interesting joy from morning to night. She never caused trouble, only gave happiness.

Now Adrienne arrived on the scene. At four months of age, she was very much a part of everything. We liked to sit her in an infant seat in the middle of the kitchen table where all the goings on were so she would be entertained. When she laughed, her smile lit up the entire house. Jimmie and I were again full of hope.

How strange the human mind is! We rebounded from the depths of despair to actually being able to think Adrienne could possibly be cured of hydrocephalus. As bright as she was, she just might live a normal life if the shunt continued to work. Adrienne's head hadn't enlarged very much, and she didn't have long intervals of increased pressure bouts that could weaken her body. Our expectations grew daily.

Jimmie and I now had fun with our children in a new way. As parents, Jimmie and I always marveled at the obvious difference in rearing a girl. Although Jim had been ill, he was obviously a boy in whatever he did.

Jeanne was all female. With fingernail polish on and lipstick to match, she clumped around all day wearing my high-heeled shoes. Her conversations were a delight, and we liked seeing her grow and develop.

Some of my happiest times were when the four of us played in the bed in the mornings and on the weekends. On one of those occasions, Jeanne announced, "I want seventeen children when I'm a mother!"

After reflecting for a moment, she remembered she would have to prepare breakfast for them and added, "No, maybe I could fix enough breakfast for ten. Ten is enough!"

One of Jimmie's brothers had ten children, and his sister had nine. There were other families of ten in town as well as one family with thirteen children. Thibodaux was about ninety-eight percent Catholic, and these large families attest to the fact that the Catholic religion was practiced scrupulously. In conversations, friends would laugh and say, "Well, maybe the eighth child will be the one to get me to Heaven. Who knows?"

Jeanne enjoyed seeing these large families with all the commotion and excitement that accompanies so many people in one house. I, too, was fascinated at how much fun it was to visit big families.

Seeing my friends continuing to become pregnant every year made me more conscious of practicing birth control. I knew I'd given birth to my last child. I was totally committed to prevent bringing any more sick children into the world.

That Christmas, Jeanne was asked to represent the Blessed Mother in a procession to be held at midnight Mass. The church was packed. Jimmie and I were seated in about the tenth row. Because of the crowd, the ushers came to the end of each row and signaled one row at a time to file out to receive communion instead of the usual practice of everyone going up as they wished. Jimmie and I had to stand up to let people pass to and from the aisle.

I felt uncomfortable going to Mass and not going up to Communion. The Catholic church had just changed the fasting rules. To receive Communion previously, one had to fast from midnight. The time had now been decreased to one hour. When a person didn't go to the altar to receive the sacrament in the past, one surmised that person needed coffee or some other sustenance before church time. I'm sure I was more conscious of not going to Communion than anyone else was. I'm sure most churchgoers didn't look around to see what others were doing. But in a rural town where everyone knows everyone else, I couldn't help but wonder if they were wondering about me. I felt the stares, real or imagined.

Yes, I felt bad, but even worse was my heartbreak at being denied the sacrament when I yearned for Jesus' body and blood. If sacrifice is pleasing to God, the sacrifice we made that night surely must have been noted. As I knelt, I argued with myself, *I want more children. I'm practicing birth control because I know it's my duty. I've tried all the methods approved by the Catholic Church, but those methods don't eliminate the possibility of my having another sick child. I'm not going to take that chance.*

I felt very close to God in the midnight hour and felt sure He understood, but I felt no signs of His encouragement.

I continued attending daily Mass when possible. Nearly everyone who attends daily Mass receives Holy Communion, so I felt strange and abandoned as I remained in my pew. The only way I could circumvent this sense of alienation was to change churches often, to vary the hours I attended Mass, and to sit in different areas in the church.

I'm sure no one was conscious Jimmie and I weren't communicants, but at the same time, I somehow believed they were. People were also quite aware we had sick children, and I didn't want to be a source of scandal. Truthfully, I feel I prayed more fervently than ever because I yearned deeply for all to be straight in God's sight.

Chapter Nineteen

Adopting Our Son

During the past year, Jimmie had spent long hours every night preparing for the American Board of Oral Surgery Certification Exam. Two years of limited private practice were required before he'd be eligible to take this exam. The percentage of people who passed wasn't very high. If one were well prepared, the written portion went very smoothly. The oral portion was the most dreaded part.

Having five separate divisions, the test was administered at the Drake Hotel in Chicago, Illinois. Each candidate went alone into a hotel room where two examiners quizzed him for half a day, a humbling experience for almost every candidate. Naturally, it would have been easier to ignore taking the exam, but Jimmie would never have allowed himself to make that choice. He prepared for a year, and on March 15 — the Ides of March — he took the exam. Weeks passed before he received the good news he'd passed. He laughed when he got the notice; not all great men fall on the Ides of March. I was happy something had gone right for him.

I'm not sure when the thought was first mentioned, but Jimmie casually commented one day, "Since we should have no more children and know how indefinite Adrienne's life expectancy is, maybe we should consider adopting a child. If we don't, Jeanne might eventually be an only child."

We were convinced Jeanne would be happier with more children in our home because almost everyone she knew had plenty of brothers and sisters. We certainly had enough love to offer another child as well as a happy home life. Knowing much time was required for the adoption process, we asked a priest friend to talk to Catholic Charities for us.

Much to our surprise, he returned in a few days with a dejected look. Catholic Charities advised, "Leave that couple alone. Just play down the idea of adopting a baby because those particular parents are surely emotionally unstable after having four children with hydrocephalus."

We couldn't believe this! There hadn't been an interview, and no effort had been made on their part to know us better or see what kind of home we could provide. We couldn't help but wonder if the organization had been misnamed since charity means love and compassion. This rejection still bothers me a little, but Jimmie still has a special place in his heart for the organization he calls, "All Catholic, no charity."

In the face of this setback, we became more determined. That failure only emphasized the vacancy in our home that could be filled by a child.

Hugh and Doris Hawthorne, a family living in our community who had adopted thirteen children, were very devoted to the Irish people. Their first two children had been adopted through normal channels in the United States, but the other eleven had been brought over from Ireland.

This couple had gone to an orphanage in Ireland many times, selected their baby, taken care of the necessary paperwork, and flown home. They knew a priest in Ireland who spent much of his spare time helping these babies find appropriate parents and happy homes in America. It was only natural Jimmie should inquire about the procedure involved in trying to find a baby in Ireland who needed a home. They suggested we contact Father Peter Shields, tell him of our situation, and ask if he'd help us qualify as adoptive parents.

Our decision to adopt wasn't a small one. We spent

hours trying to be as wise as we could possibly be in such an unfamiliar circumstance and thought this through as thoroughly as two intelligent people could. We didn't discuss adoption with anyone except Father Shields and the parents of the thirteen adopted children.

In American adoption agencies, the social worker tries to match the child to the parents' education and to their physical attributes. In Ireland, we'd know nothing at all about the baby's background or parents. This surely would be in the hands of God.

Jimmie kept saying, "Children belonging to the same mother and father in a family are individually different – different in looks, personality and abilities. I believe environment is most important, not heredity. Anyway, if you decide to give a child who needs a home a chance in life by letting him share your home, you can't question his heritage!"

To come to terms with accepting an unknown child on faith alone took me a long time. In the United States, an unborn child is often assigned to the adoptive parents, and there's no choosing the sex. We'd been told we had a choice. The most important consideration to us was Jeanne. If we adopted a boy, there'd probably not be any competition between them. She'd be the only girl and an individual in her own right. To the best of our ability, we tried to picture the future for Jeanne in making that decision. We wanted desperately for her to be happy.

We sincerely wanted to offer a home to a boy who didn't have parents because of a strange twist of fate. In doing so, we'd give him our love, an education, a warm bed, food, and guide him to find a purpose in life that would offer him satisfaction and happiness as an adult. We'd teach him to love God by our example as well as by utilizing the proper outside teaching and training offered in the community.

We made a definite decision we'd let him be his own person to live his life without our trying to over-power him. We knew this would be hard to do, but that was a goal we would earnestly strive to accomplish. We also decided if he didn't follow what we thought were proper guidelines, we wouldn't let him ruin our lives. These decisions between us seemed very important. We have had a saying about both biological and adoptive children: "Hurt us our children can, ruin our lives they cannot."

As individuals, we thought we had a lot to offer a child. We were both college graduates. Jimmie is a professional man. We hoped we had enough experience to motivate a child to learn about the world and to want to search for knowledge. We wanted to give him warmth that would make the sharp edges of life easier for him to bear. We wanted to teach him the meaning of honor and integrity. There were so many intangibles we could give to enrich his life and to show him the importance of high ideals in life. We wanted a son, and we believed we were ready and worthy to raise one.

By adopting a child, Jimmie and I would consciously work harder to attain these goals because our adopted child would be a person who hadn't asked to live in our home. I felt an even greater responsibility in rearing an adopted child than in rearing a biological one.

Jimmie wrote a letter telling the priest in Ireland our history. We waited for a reply. Father Peter Shields told us many years later that he'd taken our letter to his mother's home. It seems she'd always served as his confidant and advisor. After hearing what Jimmie said, she commented, "Please help those people if you can. They're good people and would be good parents to a baby."

Father Shields' reply was only the first step along a new and rocky road wrought with more problems than we expected. Jimmie said he'd give birth to this child, meaning he'd spend the long hours filling out the necessary papers, writing the needed letters, and gathering the necessary information. I don't believe he realized how involved or time-consuming this process would prove to be.

The Hawthornes were traveling to Ireland in March 1961, and they could lend some assistance toward the adoption through friends as well as by visiting the orphanage. The pet child in the orphanage located near Dublin was a three-month-old little boy with blue eyes and red hair — a typical Irish lad. Father Shields had also visited the orphanage and agreed this boy was the ideal one for us. Now we'd begin the long wait for permission to bring him to the United States.

Irish officials had a regulation that no babies could leave Ireland until they were a year old. This allowed Jimmie nine months to complete the overwhelming amount of paper work. When the Hawthornes brought a picture of the boy back to us, we immediately fell in love with him. One could almost see his boundless energy in this tiny snapshot.

Ireland required a social worker's report on our home, and we also had to be endorsed by, of all organizations, Catholic Charities! After our last experience with the New Orleans organization, we weren't sure just how we'd go about getting this accomplished. Father Ropollo, who'd helped us so far, had a close priest friend who knew Bishop Greco of the Archdiocese of Alexandria, the same diocese in which Benita Ann and Annette's home was located. We'd been faithful to the home, visiting on all parent days as well as many extra times during the year. We'd made donations. Our family and friends had also given generously through the years. We knew the bishop was aware of our family problems, so we hoped he'd answer our request for help.

Our other big worry was a new Irish law that permitted adoption only if we had only one other child in the home. We did — Jeanne, who was healthy. But we also had Adrienne, and our two other sick children were in the total-care home in Clarks. We needed an affidavit saying we had only one child.

Father Ropollo, Jimmie and I looked very calm the morning we departed for Alexandria to ask Bishop Greco for the favor, but inside the facade, each of us had quite a few anxieties. I kept telling myself that if we could work this out, it was God's will. If we couldn't, then that, too, was God's will. By this time, however, Jimmie and I wanted very much to have the little redhead in the picture come share his life with us.

Bishop Greco put us at ease immediately with his magnetism, goodness, and perception. Instantly, he digested our problem and discovered a solution. He was a gracious, loving man, and his eyes laughed when he said what we needed to hear, "Sometimes we have to forget certain facts, but one fact is true. You do have only one healthy child. We don't have to comment on the other three children. We'll just say you have one healthy child."

As lunch was served in his formal dining room, I looked around at the chandeliers and lovely pieces of furniture in the room, thinking of all the lonely meals this dynamic man must eat by himself because of the dictates of his lofty position. He told us grand stories as we ate, one particularly touching me.

When Bishop Greco was a child, Mother Seaton passed by him one day on the busy sidewalks of New Orleans and stopped. She put her hand on his head, saying to a companion, "One day, this boy will be a bishop." Many years later, Bishop Charles Greco attended the canonization of Mother Seaton as a saint of the Roman Catholic Church.

When the bishop drove with us to St. Mary's at Clarks for a visit, we were privileged to witness the love that shone from his face as he spoke to each of the children. His presence created joy and happiness as we moved among the rooms. He called each person by name, asking each a personal question, and waiting with interest and patience for their answers. There was no doubt they loved and trusted him. We knew he'd follow through in helping us give a home to a child who needed parents to offer him love.

The requirement that seemed most difficult was having nuns who served the role of social workers come into our home to look us over. We enjoyed sharing our home with friends and family, but this was different. This time the guests would be observing everything we did, listening carefully to our conversation, and analyzing us in order to make written statements as to our suitability for adopting a child. The ordeal also touched our pride.

I met the three nuns at the New Orleans airport and drove them to Thibodaux. In the hour-and-a-half drive, I felt they began to know me rather well, maybe too well. We served them lunch, walked them through our home, and drove them around Thibodaux. I guess Jimmie was even more miserable than I. He didn't like being observed. I could see him squirming under their watchful eyes. The time seemed extremely long, tiring and boring.

Jeanne saved the day and made them think our home would be a grand place for anyone to come and live as she entertained and charmed them with her laughs and smiles. Maybe they reasoned that any child that well mannered, well behaved, and lovable must prove her parents could rear another as well. Of course, we couldn't tell Jeanne what was going on; in fact, no one else knew.

A few days later, we received a letter saying we'd passed the examination! Now, we'd just have to wait until December 1961 for our new baby to become an Irish Cajun.

*****

Jeanne was to be four in September. I wanted this to be an extra special day, so I decided to have the merry-go-round truck for her party. Former neighbors in New Orleans had often hired it, and the children loved the musical ride. I had a terrible time persuading the owner in New Orleans to make the trip to Thibodaux. He finally relented. I had D.H. Holmes Department Store send a large cake in the shape of Jeanne's birthday number to complete the birthday party décor. Having invited all Jeanne's cousins and classmates to the party, I loved standing aside watching them have fun.

We had spent so many hours seeing children suffer that we tried to make the most of the fun times. I also felt that each time we could do extra special things for Jeanne, we should because there would be times when I appeared to be doing very special things for Adrienne because of her uncertain illness.

*****

Jimmie was invited to join a gourmet club that had been in existence a few years. There were eight members, only men. I was thrilled! This meant I could prepare all the fancy courses and have a reason to learn more about food preparation from both foreign and domestic kitchens. Because the first meal we served was Armenian, we had a whole baked lamb. This club offered another diversion to add to my list as I constantly looked for interesting ways to enrich our time so we wouldn't feel sorry for ourselves.

Another time-consuming interest on my list was the civic club I had joined before we moved to Thibodaux. Twenty-five ladies met once a month from September to May. Besides just enjoying one another's company, we had a project we went all out for one Saturday each year — a card luncheon. The proceeds were used to aid the mentally handicapped children in Thibodaux.

Because of my dietetic background, I was chairman of the food committee. Each year, this luncheon was held at a local nightclub. We were able to prepare the bridge tables in a very attractive manner on the club floor, using flowers and colorful cloths. The food, however, had to be served from a liquor storeroom. The luncheon offered our members quite a few challenges, but all the effort each year made us grow closer in friendship.

*****

Jimmie and I were outgrowing our home. The time I had dreamed of and looked forward to was finally here — time to design and build our own home. During all those years of marriage, we had at leisure times ridden up and down Bayou Lafourche looking for an appropriate building site. Our first criteria was to have one live oak tree that could spread its big branches in beauty, offering inviting shady vistas. In years gone by, Bayou Lafourche was the only mode of transportation, so all the houses faced the bayou, and the property was divided into narrow strips of land stretching from the waterway far back to the drainage canals. Most of the land belonged to the same families since the days of the Spanish land grants, and many of the people were quite reluctant to part with their inheritance. However, after much perseverance and searching on Jimmie's part, we found a fifty-acre plot about two miles from the city of Thibodaux with five glorious oak trees enhancing it. A general store and two small houses were on the site, but if we moved those three buildings, we would have a perfect spot on which to build our dream.

During those months of nausea at the beginning of my pregnancies, I spent endless hours drawing floor plans, so Jimmie and I already knew what we needed and wanted for a livable house. We both liked the old southern colonial style best and knew such a house would never go out of style along a bayou where so many columned houses had stood since the eighteenth century.

We hired an architect and even had a special model created to be sure the columns and roof were in the right proportions. Ten columns weighing two tons each would be across the front with one column dropping back on the left side. We drew numerous plans, but the front door always ended up off-center. Jimmie particularly appreciates symmetry, but we finally convinced him the off-center door added character.

We searched for old brick and were lucky enough to find an old building in St. Louis, Missouri, being demolished. These bricks were shipped down the Mississippi River to New Orleans and then to Thibodaux by truck. Among these bricks were carved decorative ones that had beautified the front of that building built in St. Louis so many years ago.

We wanted the front of the house to be white and the old bricks to be utilized in the fireplace and in the rear gallery floor and columns. Because this would be where we'd live most of our waking hours, we wanted those bricks to give those areas ambiance. I chose large-paned windows across the back so we'd enjoy the yard and the cane fields from the interior.

Immense native pecan trees graced our private back yard.

Because of Adrienne's condition, we wanted to live downstairs. No matter how well she progressed, climbing steps to her bedroom would prove too much for her. Of course, we wanted our bedroom near hers, and the other children should be near us, also. For the present, we planned to finish an upstairs guest room, leaving a large attic roughed in until a time when it could be used. We decided against building a formal living room, having looked at many homes where formal living rooms were beautifully furnished but never used. Therefore, we built a great room we could all enjoy.

Thibodaux's master builder won the construction bid and began building our home in July 1962, losing only one day because of rain. He would complete Beaux Chenes plantation thirteen months later.

Friends who'd built homes had warned us construction can be very trying to a husband and wife. Many demanding decisions need to be made each day, and a couple very often ends up angry at each other. Jimmie and I decided we were going to enjoy the project in spite of what we were being told and would have no reason to argue if we sincerely worked at finding pleasure. We wanted this home to represent the love we shared. We wanted it to be a place for happiness. Both of us had always tackled jobs striving for perfection, always trying to give our all. This new endeavor wouldn't be any different. Planning and building our dream house would give us many rewarding hours.

The early days of 1961 were good ones. Having observed other mothers with their children, I now felt our lives were beginning to approach those normal ones. I was busy with a baby who from all visible evidence was developing normally and a five-year-old who was very much a charming little lady. The days seemed to run so smoothly we were lulled into complacency.

With no effort on our part, these long days were soothing. We could hear the birds in the branches of the trees. I could stretch out on the bed after lunch and hear voices of children playing in the backyard. There was time to smell the fragrance the sun and gentle wind gave to our sheets and our linen. There was time to read long, lazy books whose subject matter could be read and forgotten. I could play the old piano pieces I had once played in uneventfully carefree childhood days. The harsh memories simmered in the back of my mind, and these long, quiet days spent just in loving two children and Jimmie were over too quickly.

Adrienne's ventriculo-cardiac shunt worked well until March 9. Just days after her first birthday, her soft spot began to be full once more. Those eight happy months plummeted into fear and despair like a big rock tumbling down from the top of a mountain, landing in snow, then falling down, down the mountain, gathering speed and more snow as it became larger and larger until it crashed into a deep valley.

Enough pressure built in Adrienne's head to cause vomiting. We drove to Mercy Hospital in New Orleans, not knowing what to expect, always hoping we wouldn't have to be admitted for a lengthy stay. This time Dr. Garcia only did a ventricular puncture to drain off her excess fluid. In just two days, Dr. Garcia said we could go home. I wanted to grab Adrienne, run and yell, "Whoopee! Halleluiah!"

I must have walked faster and made a quicker exit than anyone else checking out. We were so happy to reach home again.

Because the heart shunt was different, we now were insecure with the complicated surgery. Following Adrienne's two days in the hospital, my worried thoughts came near depression. Until now we had reason to hope the heart shunt was going to win the hydrocephalus battle. The neurosurgeons thought this new surgical procedure was the answer. However, after this pressure build-up, all my anxieties returned. The long peace and quiet I'd enjoyed were slipping away.

*****

Official word came that the nuns who were sent to judge

our desirability as parents for an adopted child recommended us. Mounds of paper work had to be completed, but we now knew we were assured of getting our little boy in December when he would be a year old. We kept all of this a secret until we would hurtle the final obstacles.

Adrienne had become very strong and could hold her head up. In October, after seven months with no increased pressure indications, back to New Orleans we had to go. Once again we were in Mercy Hospital for two days. Once again that falling rock was gathering momentum. Sure enough, one month later we entered the hospital on November 2 in real trouble. At eighteen months, one of the most adorable ages for a little girl, Adrienne went back into the dreaded operating room, and a replacement ventriculo-cardiac shunt procedure was performed.

In addition to the sick feeling we had about another serious surgery, we felt disappointment seeing her suffer a setback in her progress of developing normally. Insignificant as that worry might seem in the light of serious surgery, we were still human and couldn't prevent the human side of that drama from entering our minds.

But seeing Adrienne's laughing sparkling eyes, her big smile, and her non-knowing attitude, we could concentrate on keeping her happy. That was our secret to showing a happy outlook when we were discouraged. Adrienne's hourly happiness was somehow temporarily more important than what was happening inside her body. That seemed to be the most logical way for us to look at the problem since we had no control over her bodily development. Besides, we had to protect our own sanity at crucial times.

At eighteen months of age, Adrienne knew us. Because there was no getting a nurse to stay with her, I moved into the hospital. The surgery was long and tedious as always, but her shunt was functioning beautifully. Through all our children's surgeries, we'd never had an immediate post-operative result like this. We were in the hospital only twelve days, and then we were back home. This seemed too good to be true!

Adrienne's head had been shaved, but by the time we reached home on November 15, a little blonde fuzz had begun to grow. When her eyes lit up, her shaved head was quickly forgotten – she was beautiful. We had a grand reunion with Jeanne and were looking forward to a new adventure. Our baby boy would be leaving Ireland after his first birthday on December 5.

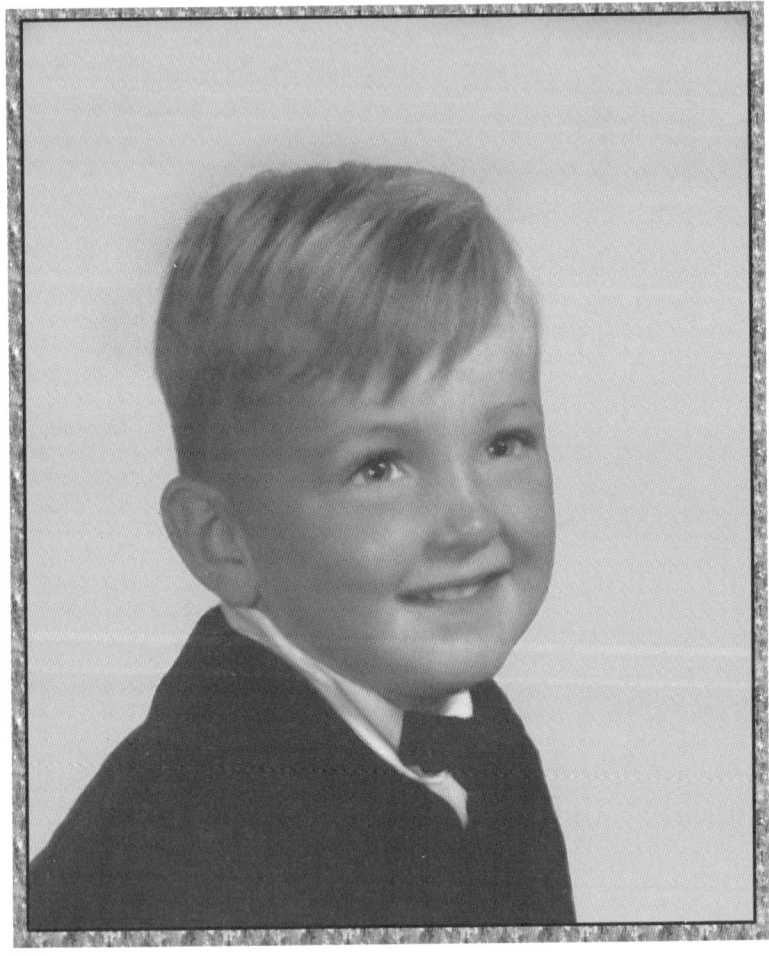

Robert James Peltier

Chapter Twenty

Robert's Arrival

*O*ur paying for a round trip passage for an Irish nurse to bring the baby from Dublin was the most convenient way to get our baby to the United States. Because the orphanage in Ireland was very poor, we sent money ahead to provide new clothes for him so he'd at least have a coat, pants, and shoes. Since we were to meet him in New York, we took a few jars of baby food, some diapers, and a baby bottle with us to nourish him before we reached Thibodaux. Even though his arrival was imminent, we decided not to tell anyone for there was always the possibility something could go wrong.

To meet a year-old boy who was from that moment to become our son was a strange sensation initially. Feelings of happiness were mixed with plenty of uneasiness. Jimmie and I had seen a picture of our new baby when he was three months of age, but other than that, we knew nothing about him. All was being done through our faith in God.

I was scared as we waited for the Irish airline's plane to land. The ground agents knew of our impending international exchange, so they let us stand on the roof of the building with a high wall around to watch people descend the steps from the plane.

Everyone deplaned, but no one came off carrying a baby. After a time lapse, all the plane's crew, pilots, stewardesses, and a nurse with a baby finally came down the steps. From our high vantage point, we couldn't see the baby's face. All we could see was a baby in the nurse's arms.

We went down to wait outside customs until all the crew was cleared. At last, the courier walked through the doors and handed our baby to us. Jimmie handed her the payment envelope and went to fill out some required papers and to collect our new baby's passport from the airline.

My new baby and I were alone. I had no idea what he liked to eat or what toys amused him. I was holding a twenty-five pound little boy dressed in an adorable blue wool suit. His hair looked as if someone had put a soup bowl over it to cut it. My only thought was he must be frightened. But he was not – he was so good. There were no tears, just two big clear blue eyes staring at me.

Jimmie and I had chosen a name for our new baby. Since our first son had been a junior, we didn't want to use that name again. So we decided to turn the name around. Instead of James Robert, we called our new son Robert James. Here he was in completely strange surroundings among strange people with strange accents, and now he had to answer to a new name. Our son had literally been transplanted from one continent and put down in another world. When my mind began to clear about this, I tried to make him feel welcome. After all, we had to get to know one another.

As Robert and I were becoming acquainted, Jimmie arrived with a taxi that took us from Irish to Delta Airlines. With Jimmie present, we were all three more at ease as Jimmie's gift of gab got us through the first anxious hour and we boarded our plane to New Orleans.

Most of our flight was spent watching Robert stare at his new parents. Finally, I decided to feed him. He sat very still with his hands in his lap and opened his mouth when I put the spoon to his lips. He ate as long as I fed him and didn't show any signs of wanting more when I had finished. If we put him in one position, he would stay there until we placed him somewhere else. There was no wiggling, moving, or reaching like most babies. He was very well-behaved and obviously had received a good measure of discipline at his former home.

When we reached Thibodaux about midnight, we foolishly awakened Jeanne and Adrienne. We explained who the redhead was and that the two of them now had a new little brother. They accepted it all very nonchalantly and played with him into the early morning hours. When time came to go to sleep, no one would get in bed, so the five of us slept together that night in our bed.

A good portion of the next day was spent announcing the news of Robert's arrival to our family and our closest friends. Soon the greeters came, but Robert wouldn't let anyone hold him except Jimmie and me, although he did make friends with Jeanne and Adrienne. He liked his new bed, and when he awakened each morning, he'd play in it until someone came to see about him. His conditioned behavior lasted about a week until he realized that if he called or made noises, someone answered. He did suck his first two fingers on his left hand, but we decided that as soon as he became secure with his new surroundings and with us, this would cease, and it did.

Robert fit right in with our household meal and sleeping schedule, so having one more baby to care for didn't upset our routine at all. But Robert had so much natural energy that we had to watch him every minute to make sure he didn't hurt himself.

Jeanne's life wasn't disturbed by our new addition. She was fascinated with Robert. Clearly, she had never seen anybody move around so fast and get into such unusual places. She liked all the stir Robert created as he enlivened our household. Everyone Jeanne knew had plenty of sisters and brothers, so I had the impression she felt more normal having another member added to our family. Neither of the girls showed any jealousy and took Robert right in stride.

Because Adrienne could stand up alone now, we hoped she would walk before long. Jeanne was entering kindergarten and offered the stabilizing joy that acted as a catalyst to our happiness. We had Robert, and soon there would be another boy.

After Robert had been with us a few months, Jimmie wrote to Father Shields stating that if another outstanding baby boy became available, we'd like to have another child live with us. Jimmie felt two boys close together in age could be friends and enjoy growing up together. He'd always wished for a brother near his age. We also felt that if they became disturbed in their teenage years about being adopted, the two would have each other to discuss their mutual problem.

Sure enough, Father Shields called us in July to say a little boy would be available who had been born on October 8, 1961. This meant the boys would be ten months apart and even begin school the same year. This second boy wouldn't be able to leave Ireland until October 1962, but we had to begin all the paper work again. Because we'd already been approved by the Alexandria diocese Catholic Charities, the procedure this time wasn't as involved. We told no one about this — only the two of us shared the excitement together.

Although very busy, our life was wonderful! Maybe God was going to let Adrienne grow up to be a normal little girl. Her shunt was functioning, and she was developing both physically and mentally. I still found myself trying to comprehend what God had in mind, although by now, I should have learned I had no such expertise. God always had His plan, and I, while praying, "Thy will be done," still had to struggle to really mean the prayer and not try to predict the future.

Because Adrienne's surgery had produced the desired results quickly, she suffered little regression. She could sit up and, at last, was now able to hold up her head. Usually we moved her from one spot to another in her carry seat and used the stroller to take her outside for walks. Sadly, there was no way she could crawl with her heavy head. But she didn't know the difference because we usually anticipated her every desire so well and she directed us to where she wished to be with noises and sounds mothers can interpret.

My only heartache was we had essentially been excommunicated from the Catholic Church. Because Jimmie and I practiced birth control, we still were unable to receive Communion. Surely God must have understood. We were adopting two babies, which proved we wanted more children. We were only preventing other hydrocephalics from coming into the world. How could this be wrong? As usual, no signs from Heaven were forthcoming.

Benita Ann and Annette were as happy as possible in Clarks. We visited every few weeks, and Jimmie's father went a few times a year, also. The girls were well, always clean, and from what we could observe, they were two special ones with the nuns and staff. The nurses seemed to also be attracted to them in a special way. Both girls had pleasant expressions on their faces, almost looked angelic and laughed a lot for no reason.

I still spent too much time thinking about Jim. His not being confirmed before his death continued to bother me. Each sacrament we receive on earth gives us a greater degree of happiness in Heaven, so it bothered me his cup couldn't run over. I knew his not being given this sacrament shouldn't have been such a burden to me. Because I didn't intend to let this happen again, I asked that Benita Ann and Annette be confirmed. They each had one person who gave them extra care, so these young ladies stood as their sponsors. Once Benita Ann and Annette were confirmed, I felt we'd done everything we could for their afterlife with God, and all had been fulfilled with them.

Knowing how quickly Jim had died and having three other children with hydrocephalus, I always kept a black dress for funerals in my closet. To realize I had to be so constantly prepared for death at the age of thirty was terribly eerie to me. I thought too often of that black dress hanging in the back of my closet.

No matter how full a person keeps a day, each hour provides

too much time to think. Busy work doesn't still the mind. I wondered about Jim over and over, and I dwelled on Benita Ann and Annette's health. No matter how many times I told myself we made the right decision placing them in a special home, I always wondered if we had, indeed, done the correct thing. Was that truly the will of God, or had we taken it upon ourselves to make a decision that didn't please Him?

Being optimistic by nature, I tried to think positively, but with previous heartaches, with Jim's death, and with Benita Ann and Annette's meningitis, I was haunted by my thoughts. I watched Adrienne's development with apprehension. If only I could receive Holy Communion, I knew I would feel better. I would be in childbearing age for fifteen more years. How could I manage everything if I were unable to participate in the sacraments of the church for so long a time? Jimmie expressed our predicament as being able to be on the team, but not being allowed to play in the game.

Chapter Twenty-One

✝

Traumatic Changes

*J*n November 1962, Pope John V called the Ecumenical Council to order in Rome, Italy. Suddenly far-reaching, visible signs of change came to the Catholic church. The mysticism I had experienced for so long was suddenly lost when the altar was moved forward toward the congregation so the priest could face us as he said Mass. The Mass was now being said in English, not in Latin as it had been for centuries. The liturgy that had been used for hundreds of years was rewritten.

At St. Joseph Church, the beautiful marble altar rails were removed, as they were all across the country. Catholics now received communion by standing in line to receive the Host and were no longer required to abstain from eating meat on Friday. The Lenten period which used to be a time of fasting and penance for us was all but eliminated. No longer did the church enforce the required penances. We were now given the opportunity to make our own choice of a private penance.

New ideas were being revealed about the sacrament of Penance. We were discouraged from frequent use of the confessional. There was now a new way to go to Confession. We no longer said, "Bless me, Father, for I have sinned It has been two weeks since my last confession. These are my sins, etc."

Instead, confession was more personal. We were to state

our station in life, whether we were single, married, or had children, or whatever. Then we could better describe our sins, and the priest could better understand the sins and offer more positive help. We no longer recited the *Act of Contrition* in the confessional. Instead, it was said in a pew after the priest had given us penance and granted absolution. Confessionals remained almost empty as the long lines that had been there on Saturdays and before daily Mass disappeared. Hours scheduled for confession were reduced on Saturdays. I wondered how a custom that had remained prevalent for so many centuries could suddenly change so completely.

I wondered about indulgences, the doctrine I'd found particularly difficult to accept when I became a Catholic. I'd been taught that each of us would spend time in Purgatory after death for the sins we had committed on earth. For instance, if I blessed myself with Holy Water after Mass and Communion within two weeks after receiving the sacrament of Confession, sixty days were removed from my time in Purgatory after my death. I was now being told from the pulpit that unless I'd committed a serious sin, there was no need for me to go to confession often as every devout Catholic had always done in the past. Most indulgent acts required they be performed within two weeks of confession. I used to go to confession once a month to gain an indulgence at any time. Had all these promises disappeared?

After the Ecumenical Council, our priests seemed to have self-proclaimed new freedoms to write and speak about any subject they chose. Most of the clergy and religious seemed to savor these changes as a chance to think on their own and to offer new and exciting things to do rather than the staid procedures and rituals. I began to hear there never was a Garden of Eden with Adam and Eve; Genesis was a story passed down through the years to explain sin. One by one, teachings Catholics had had engrained since childhood were destroyed. Nuns put away their graceful habits for street clothes, no longer being readily recognized as religious sisters. I learned Saint Christopher was no longer the protector we thought him to be for travels. Rote prayers said over and over were no longer fashionable for Catholics. This idea even attacked the foundation of something deeply Catholic, the Rosary.

Music and prayer in unison began to fill the once quiet time for prayer and meditation during Mass. Our congregation received lessons in singing before every Mass as the old hymns gave way to swinging new musical beats with equally unfamiliar words. Unkempt youth with guitars were at the altar. As I attended different Catholic churches, I was likely to find each service different from pastor to pastor. Our Catholic church was no longer one.

About the same time as the changes in the church, the birth control pill burst on the scene. Every paper, magazine, and talk show proclaimed its wonders. Catholic parishes all over heard about this priest or that priest who had given someone permission to use the pill. About half gave permission and half didn't. This was all very confusing to me. I wondered, "What about Pope Paul VI's *Humanae Vitae Encyclical*. Is this being ignored?"

I read; I kept up; but there'd been no warning the Catholic Church I'd come to love so much would begin to be very different. The windows Pope John XXIII wanted to open to let in fresh air seemed to be admitting a hurricane.

I looked around at others who attended Mass as I did. These changes had such an impact on my life I couldn't believe others weren't as deeply confused. I thought the elderly church members would be greatly displeased, but discussions with them made it clear they were adjusting with the passage of time. It was almost like watching something pure become tainted.

Maybe this change was accented in my life because Jimmie felt it even more than I did. He'd grown up in the Catholic Church. The church and the ritual of the Mass were a way of life with him. They symbolized something unchanging in life. Nothing else remains static, but to him, the rock of the Catholic Church would never change.

There were disgruntled discussions amongst our friends, but I saw no one take this as hard as Jimmie. Already Jimmie wondered if God had turned His back on him with the constant "no" to our prayers, but now he was finding the place where he worshipped and the way he worshipped had changed drastically.

I watched a bitterness beginning to take root. And in the middle of so much confusing changes, we still couldn't even go to Communion. I believe if we hadn't had children for whom to set the example, Jimmie might have discontinued going to church altogether.

I spent hours trying to analyze why these changes disturbed Jimmie so much more than everyone else. He'd been an altar boy in his youth. His mother told me that as a young boy, he'd built an altar in his room and spoke of having a vocation. He had catechism taught to him year after year. With his bright mind, he'd learned his rote and philosophical lessons well.

If he'd been a man who had married, had several healthy children, and lived a so-called normal life, he'd have attended Mass every Sunday, attended Mass daily during Lent, followed the church laws and had a normal man-to-God relationship. Instead, he had five children, four of whom had hydrocephalus. This was a devastating religious crisis to him. His only hope was God, and he'd turned to the church and God to help him.

There was no other hope but God. There was absolutely nothing Jimmie and I as human beings could do to make our children well. Most things a person desires in life can be obtained by hard work, either physically or mentally. No amount of personal effort on our part could cure hydrocephalus. With money, a person can buy goods that can contribute to his happiness. No amount of money can buy health.

We were desperate. Our hope lay with the power of God. Jimmie turned to Him body and soul and begged. Along with the begging, he did penance by depriving himself of small daily pleasures. At times when it would have been possible for him to rest or relax, he went to church. He abstained from food he enjoyed eating to offer penance to God. I often thought that if he could have worn a rough rope around his waist as St. Francis did, he'd have made that sacrifice. In spite of all his prayers and all his penance, he felt he was trapped and helpless.

I always felt that to Jimmie, God was the church, and the church was God. Jimmie had spent hours each day at church on his knees praying since our first child had been born in 1954. During those eight years, the church had been the same as it had always been when he was a child, and God would hear and answer his prayers and requests. But now Jimmie had lost one son at five years of age. He knew it was only a matter of time until two more of his children would die. Now he was praying desperately to God to cure the fourth child. The one thing Jimmie had depended upon to remain the same when his life was falling down around him was the church. That church seemed to be betraying him and crumbling.

We began to notice priests going out more often to cocktail parties. Priests and nuns began leaving their religious orders to marry. Brothers of the Sacred Heart who had taught Jimmie, men who were so dear to him, began to depart in droves. At first, Jimmie was shocked and hurt by these changes, but gradually, he became bitter.

Of course, there was an associated factor. Jimmie now always seemed to get a "no" answer from God. It was as if he had drawn a cloak of bitterness around himself in order to protect himself from being hurt again. He'd act the same outwardly, but inside, he wasn't going to let himself be vulnerable again.

All this happened slowly. The only person left who hadn't changed, hadn't hurt him, and who really knew how much hurt he suffered was me. I was the only one the tight protective circle had not shut out. Jeanne wasn't old enough yet. She was his young child he loved. That protective barrier didn't exclude her.

177

Now I prayed for something else. I prayed I could be the person to meet Jimmie's needs so someday with enough love from me and enough time to soften his hurt, he could again return to his love for God. All I could do was love him and wait.

When he spoke of not going to church, I tried to laugh and say, "Oh, no, you're not getting out of this! You always said you converted me because of your saintly example. (This was his private joke.) We had all these sick children because of my promise to the Catholic Church. You're not pulling out on me now!" That would end the conversation, and he'd keep coming to church with us.

With the passage of time, I forced myself to adjust as well as I could to all these changes because I saw there was no turning back for the Church. The windows had been nailed open. I loved God, and if this was to be the future of the church, I would have to go along with it. I tried to read and understand what was happening. I could even enjoy the new music that turned Jimmie off completely. Though he tried to cover it up for my sake, he couldn't hide his displeasure from me.

One day, Jimmie told me, "I can never ask God for anything again." And he meant it. Those beautiful thoughts about God he had written while Jim was first sick, which now seemed like another lifetime ago, weren't the thoughts he now had. I could tell he wanted to stand face to face with his Creator and have the opportunity to plead his case. It is difficult to be told "no" by God at every turn, especially when your little child is suffering. That is the worst of it all. We learned a lesson well. There are things much worse than death.

Chapter Twenty-Two

David Charles

October 8, 1962, came. Our baby waiting in Ireland was now a year old, but this time, the Irish bureaucratic machine had slowed. Unimportant delays had obstructed the final clearance for our son's departure, and he wouldn't be allowed to come until the red tape had been cut. Each month we thought word would come with the date of his arrival in New York, but the months dragged on. Finally, we were told to come at the end of April 1963. Because he'd assisted us so much in the adoption proceedings, we decided to invite Father Ropollo to fly with us to New York.

Father Ropollo, Jimmie and I left Louisiana to go meet our second adopted son a few days early. We wanted to find a Madonna to place in a specially prepared niche on the staircase of our home under construction. That search for just the right statue was interesting. In a special section of Manhattan devoted to church needs, we found the perfect Madonna carved of wood. I was still working on my devotion to Mary, and I hoped this would help.

I'd always found traveling with a priest exciting because we were able to go with him each day to fulfill his requirement of saying daily Mass. Father Ropollo had chosen a private altar located behind the main altar at St. Patrick's Cathedral, so we went to Mass each morning with him. Father knew but never mentioned our reason for not receiving Communion.

We had fun eating at Mama Leoni's. One should always go there with a priest. The collar truly worked miracles. There was no standing in lines; the best tables were offered; and the service was impeccable.

As the three of us went to await the arrival of the airplane bringing our newest son, an announcement was made that inclement weather had forced the plane to land in Montreal, Canada, for the night. We were sorely disappointed as we scurried to find rooms at the airport to be there first thing in the morning.

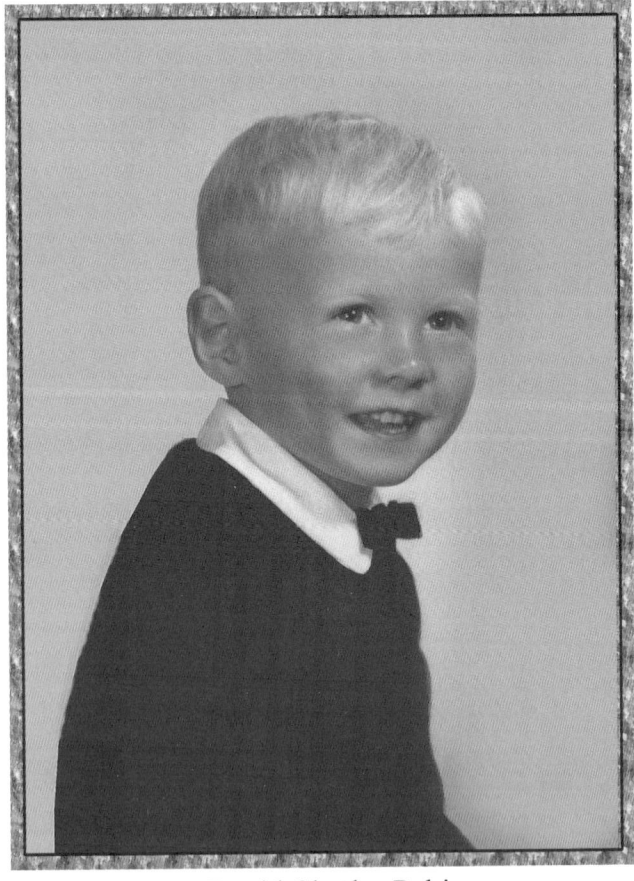

David Charles Peltier

Bright and early the following morning, we were at the airport waiting for the plane. A male nurse carrying a very blonde baby was one of the first people down the steps of the plane. Our having gone through this once before didn't make the second time any less of a moving experience, but this time there were three of us to try to entertain our new son and make him welcome. It's hard to imagine the emotions involved with his being taken from familiar surroundings, flying with strangers across the Atlantic, spending the night in Montreal with strangers, and then being given to three more strangers.

Our new baby clung to me. I suppose he'd known only females, the nuns in Ireland, as he held on tightly. He wouldn't get down on the floor. His legs would straighten out, but he refused to attempt to stand. He didn't cry, but we could see fear in his blue eyes. The extra night in Montreal must have been a traumatic time for him. If the plane had come in on time, he would have been less frightened. Fortunately, we departed from New York early in the morning and were able to reach Thibodaux in record time.

On May 1, 1963, our new son arrived in a new home with a new family. Because he had had nothing familiar in his environment for about sixty hours, I tried to hold him and rock him a lot to offer the love he so needed.

Being around other children helped, but he still clung to me, and he wouldn't put his feet on the floor. I became so concerned I insisted Jimmie call the Irish home to inquire. They assured him all was well; our little boy could walk and ordinarily was a relaxed baby. Jeanne even dressed up like a nun with a white cover over her head to make him feel more at home. After a few days, David began to walk and to join in our family life.

We decided to name him David Charles because David was my favorite boy's name from the Bible since I was a child, and Charles after Bishop Charles Greco.

Here we were again with four children, and three very near the same age. Adrienne was eight months older than Robert, who was ten months older than David. In essence, the three were constant companions. Adrienne called them "my boys" as soon as she could talk. I never let the three of them interfere with the things Jeanne participated in since she was older.

Meal times and naptimes remained unchanged even with our new addition. I simply think of this time as a very busy one. There were many diapers to change, many prayers to say at night, and much food to be cooked and served. Thank goodness, I had good help. Thank God for Jimmie and his all out interest. We had Jeanne, Adrienne, Robert and David to rear. Jimmie didn't change toward them. I believe it was God and the adult world that had hurt him, certainly not his children. Our lives were in a rushed turmoil after having been so tranquil. I resolved then and there that we had acted on good faith. I was in this all the way!

*****

Construction on our new home continued to progress. How thankful I was our four children would move into their home at such a young age. They'd really grow up in that house, and I hoped they'd have happy memories.

Beaux Chenes, our new home, was completed in just over a year. We moved in on August 12, 1963. Jeanne had her very own bedroom. Adrienne was to share a room with Jeanne, but she preferred sleeping with "my boys." Robert and David thought that was a wonderful idea. Each child chose his place to sit at the breakfast room table, and special rules regarding where food could be eaten were instituted. After our having visited the house so many times during its construction, our children were right at home when we moved in, and we were delighted.

I made sure we had a picture of Jesus in our home, a crucifix in each bedroom and the new statue of the Blessed Mother on our staircase. The priest came to bless our home, and as so often in the past, we counted our blessings. After all our heartaches, we were much more aware when there were happy times.

Adrienne was doing well. She learned to walk, but her heavy head didn't move in synchrony with the rest of her body. So when she walked or ran, she looked different from anyone else. This wasn't something anyone else noticed, but Jimmie and I loved her so much that we spent much time just watching her. That she could walk at all was a miracle to us.

Jeanne entered second grade in September, and I was at home with my triplets. We searched for pecans in the fall. Behind our house were sugarcane fields, so from our back porch, we saw the changing scene offered by the cane fields. Every third year, a cane field is plowed under and planted with some other crop so the land can rejuvenate itself to produce cane for another three years. We saw the freshly plowed fields. We watched the cane being planted and saw its progress through fertilization and the growth period until it stood tall and willowy in the fall, ready for harvest. We spent hours watching the unusual pieces of farm machinery used to harvest the cane.

Only a wire fence separated us from horses next door, so we often strolled around the yard watching the horses. The three children and I spent many hours outside basking in the pleasure of country living.

The time finally came to teach our children all I wanted to share. I spent hours reading aloud to them. We all liked to swing in an over-sized swing on the back porch and sing. There was the gym set. I liked to give them a big push on the swing and then "let the cat die" as the swing slowed to a halt. The two boys scrambled up and zoomed down the slide over and over each day.

Jimmie and I were fortunate to live in a small town that allowed most offices to close for lunch. Happy times were spent while our children watched for Daddy to come home at noon and then again a five o'clock. We laughed constantly and enjoyed being together. The ordinary things we did were the same things other mothers, fathers, and children all over the country were doing, but this was the first time Jimmie and I were able to live this way although we had had children for nine years. I felt great joy at participating in these ordinary pastimes.

Jimmie had nicknames for all our children: the Swan was Jeanne, T-Rouge for Robert, Charlie my boy or Big Toe for David, and Lizzy Bird for Adrienne. Jimmie often called to them in French, but when he pronounced their first two names, they instantly knew he was displeased.

My days were full and happy. I still haunted the churches praying for Adrienne, Benita Ann, and Annette. I didn't spend hours trying to put my prayers into words. Rather, I made a statement like, "You know I'm here. I love you. Please help me."

I still changed churches and areas in churches to call less attention to the fact I couldn't receive Holy Communion. Then one day, while I was kneeling before Mass wishing I could go to Communion, a priest came up to me and said, "Ann, come into the confessional."

I gasped, but naturally, I hastened to follow the priest's orders. When I knelt down in the confessional, he began by saying, "You know it's all right for you to take the pill." He continued by saying priests have the power to give permission to use available methods of birth control when there is a real reason to use preventive measures. He talked to me for a long time.

It was true. People were aware of my not receiving Communion. I was bothered priests noticed my fervent devotion through the years and had been aware I always remained in the pew at communion time. This church wasn't even the main church in Thibodaux. It was an outlying one I used so people wouldn't be aware of me at Mass.

Trying not to cry, I began to tell him how sorry we were that we found it necessary to practice birth control and how I longed for the sacraments.

He said, "You don't have to explain. Everyone knows

about your sick children, and I can see your heartache."

I told him I knew priests were giving this permission, but I had never been able to bring myself to seek out one of them.

He told me again he knew I was a convert and repeated again the powers of a priest, "Whose sins you forgive are forgiven, and whose sins you retain are retained." He insisted his instructions to me were pleasing to God.

When I assured him Jimmie would never accept my taking the pill while going to Communion, he suggested Jimmie call him. But I knew that would never work, so I asked, "Is there any way you could come to our house and talk to us both?"

He was very obliging. That night he explained at length the stand of the Church in necessary cases. Jimmie had had ingrained in him that birth control should be a sin, but he conceded only because this meant so much to me. Jimmie kept saying, "What about all of those people who went to Hell because they practiced birth control?"

My only response was, "Look, this priest found us; we didn't find him. Times change. Surely it must be all right for me to take the pill. It's not something I made up."

How happy I was to return to Communion. How nice it was to enter church through the regular door on the left side of the church I'd used in the past and sit in the familiar pew on the left side of the aisle!

I decided not to look back. Once I made up my mind we were going to take the priest's suggestion, I felt we would have to change with the times. I was so happy to be back receiving the sacraments! Jimmie received the sacrament, also, but I felt sometimes he thought he was committing a worse sin by being unworthy to receive the Host.

*****

On September 1, 1963, Jeanne had a big birthday party at our new home. A horse with a little buggy for the children to ride in was the favorite of all her guests. In October David celebrated his second birthday. I asked the whole family, adults and all, to come out on Sunday since this was David's first birthday in the U.S.A. We filled a wheelbarrow with ice and cokes, had sandwiches and cakes, and everyone seemed to have fun.

Robert was three in December. Ordinarily, people think December birthdays are not as much fun as birthdays in other months because Christmas is so near, but I tried to make December 5 great for him. We decorated with crepe paper and balloons and set up a pin-the-tail-on-the-donkey game.

I was determined we'd all live a normal life. I wanted to shout, "Look, I'm normal. Look at me, I'm normal!"

We bought new Christmas decorations because we had a new house. Sending Christmas cards with family pictures was fashionable. This would be the perfect time because we had a new house and two adopted sons to include in a picture with all our children. But, sadly, we could never consider doing that because we wouldn't want to hurt Adrienne. When people saw her alone, most weren't aware of her head being larger than other children's because her personality overshadowed that. In a still photograph, the possibility for comparison with other smaller heads would have been very obvious and painful. I didn't want to create any possibility for such a comparison nor give her even the vestige of such pain.

That Christmas Santa made a big stopover and brought many presents down the new chimney of Beaux Chenes. The nice new bedrooms and large closets had room for all the toys. I felt we tried to fill empty spaces too quickly.

We went to Jimmie's parents' home for Christmas dinner. All our children could walk and find their own fun. This was the first time we had ever had a Christmas like this. Always before, we wanted to be near the child who needed us as an insurance for their fun. Now I could join the adults, enjoy some independence, and watch our children from afar, too. It was a milestone. My goodness, four children and everyone happy!

Chapter Twenty-Three

Benita Ann's Death

$\mathcal{I}$n the early hours of the morning on December 12, 1964, Jimmie and I received a long distance call from St. Mary's. Benita Ann had just died for no apparent reason from cardiac arrest. She was nine years old, had been alert for three months of her life, had never known anything about herself, and had undergone eight operations before her body was free of pain. Loving hands and voices had cared for her during her entire life.

Jimmie and I were both numb and heartbroken. Jimmie's first reaction was to call the priest at St. Joseph's. We were still searching for some kind words from one of God's representatives. As the housekeeper tried to protect the priest's sleep, Jimmie, in his inimitable way, let her know the pastor was wanted on the phone post haste. He asked the priest to make Benita Ann's funeral as simple as possible and as quickly as possible. Jimmie always found the time between his child's death and final burial unbearable.

I wanted to go straight to Clarks.

"A five-hour drive is unnecessary," the people at Clarks insisted. "There is nothing you can do. Just call the funeral home in Thibodaux and have them send the hearse for her."

Again, Jimmie and I had to wait. We always seemed to be waiting around for big heartaches. The waiting seemed

187

interminable. Only five years had passed since all our friends and relatives had come to St. Joseph's to help us through Jim's death. Now we'd have to live through another wake and funeral.

Jeanne had a beautiful soft blue velvet dress with appliquéd flowers that would fit Benita Ann, so we chose that for her burial dress. Decisions like that helped keep us busy, helped time pass.

Our faithful, wonderful family and friends came the next morning. This time, I seemed to be sleepwalking. Each thing we did brought Jim's death back so vividly. I couldn't help but wonder what must be ahead for Annette and Adrienne. I had no doubt my husband was having identical thoughts. The past, the present and the future all seemed bound together in sorrow.

By now we'd learned to think logically, but this didn't mean our emotions were stilled. The song, "the Strife is O'er, the Battle Done," seemed to fit Benita Ann's life. We felt sad for her little wasted life. In grief, once again our sorrow turned to melancholy that we had four children with such a rare, deforming birth defect. No parent can ever lose a child and ever be the same again. No one can know that hurt unless he has experienced it.

At the funeral parlor, Jimmie and I were allowed to be alone with Benita Ann before the doors opened to the public. Even in death, she was unusually beautiful. That pure, calm face still resembled what our earthly minds think an angel should look like. I regretted I had a part in bringing her into the world to suffer. I remembered the teaching of the past that when entering heaven, a soul particularly loves the parents who gave him the opportunity to be born so his soul could dwell in happiness with God forever. I hoped Benita Ann loved us even though our genes had given her a bad time here on earth.

I remembered, too, that there is no sorrow, no deformity, no tears and no pain in Heaven. Benita Ann had suffered untold pain. For months she screamed in pain because the tube in her ureter had abscessed, and she had been through all those brain surgeries. If to suffer on earth is to make our happiness in the hereafter even greater, then surely, Benita Ann must have the greatest joy God can give to someone her age.

I knew Benita Ann was in Heaven because she never learned what a sin was. She had been baptized and confirmed; therefore, she had every possible sacrament offered by the Church to someone her age.

I didn't weep or show outward emotion at her death. I couldn't believe I was reliving this kind of hurt again. I felt as if an old wound had ruptured. Memories crowded me, choking me. I felt helpless knowing I could do nothing about Benita Ann's death nor could I alter the course that lay ahead.

My mother always seemed able to do anything for me I needed. I thought I, too, would be able to make everything all right for my children. I wanted to be with them, to protect them from hurt. I wanted to be strong to make their lives happy. I had a devastating feeling when I realized once again I couldn't meet the needs of my sick children. I felt an almost savage despair. Only God could help, but He didn't seem to want.

The nuns from Clarks came to Thibodaux en masse. Knowing Benita Ann had been given true love in their care was a comfort. Minutes ticked by. We shook hands with the throngs so kind to come to the funeral home. Sometimes people insisted we go to the back of the funeral home for a coke. We accepted because we sensed this made them feel they were doing something for us. However, Jimmie and I just wanted to stand near Benita Ann's coffin, near all the beauty she offered even in death.

One curious thing both of us noticed as Jim and Benita Ann lay in their coffins — something was missing, the utter lack of vitality — the complete absence of personality   their bodies were there, but their person had flown away.

Time did pass. The White Mass of the Angels was offered again. The Church again reminded us our young innocent child was in Heaven with God this day. I found solace in rising from my pew and joining the Communion line. My being able to go to Communion had been granted just in time for Benita Ann's funeral.

Instead of having the funeral home chauffeur this time, we drove in our car, just Jeanne, Jimmie and me. Jeanne was always our hope and joy. This time I could have thrown my arms around her and hugged her.

As she sat dressed up in the back seat of the car looking out of the window, she said, "We're leading the parade. There's a parade behind us!"

We all laughed. With that laugh, we realized again we had to work at living on the bright side. Our lives required such pain and loneliness so often that we welcomed Jeanne's reminder of a normal life.

As I put away my black dress, I wondered if the styles would change before it would have to be used again. I thought about Benita Ann in Heaven with Jim. At least, they had each other. Now they could look down from Heaven and really know their earthly mother and father.

I resolved to make each deed I did each day pleasing just in case they wanted to know me better. I still wished for a sign or some way to be reassured.

Each day I said the extra *Our Father* at the end of my rosary for Jim; I now added another. I knew no better way to pay them a tribute daily. I had read that St. Theresa, the Little Flower, had appeared to someone after her death and said, "I would come back to earth and undergo all the suffering again in order to say one *Lord's Prayer* because it pleases God so immensely."

If this were true, I would do that each day for my two saints.

Chapter Twenty-Four

✝

A Happy Time

$\mathcal{W}$e had learned through the years to continue our normal activities. No matter what we felt in our hearts, we learned to put those thoughts out of view and to participate in the life around us. Since no one in Thibodaux had known Benita Ann, our mourning was completely different than if she'd lived in our home and in our town and had friends of her own here.

Jimmie was to be the Mardi Gras King of the Krewe of Chronos in Thibodaux. So many secret preparations can be made, the carnival king is chosen months ahead. Now we'd be taking leading roles in this community extravaganza taking place in March, two months after Benita Ann's funeral.

Jimmie and I certainly didn't delight in the idea of revelry, but we had other members of our family to consider. We couldn't disappoint Jimmie's parents, and my mother was planning to come to the celebration. Jeanne was old enough to enjoy the festivities, and our other three children could also have fun. I decided that although the preparations would be painful, we'd try to enjoy the event.

Mardi Gras, or Fat Tuesday, is the last day before Ash Wednesday ushers in the forty days of Lent leading to Easter. In preparation for the subdued time to come, much revelry goes on during the weeks climaxing with Mardi Gras Day. Most people associate Mardi Gras with New Orleans, but throughout South Louisiana, many other towns also host the lavish balls and the parades with cries of "Throw me something, Mister." We enjoy our celebration in Thibodaux even more because everyone here knows everyone else.

The Krewe of Chronos pageant was held at the Thibodaux Civic Center. Everyone donned their very best finery to watch the revelers dressed in elaborate costumes and see the presentation of their maids and the King and Queen. Many months had been spent making the krewe's costumes of beautiful fabrics covered with gold and silver trim, glowing pearls, plush fur, and exotic feathers. To be invited to reign as king is a great honor. Jimmie was to be the youngest king the Krewe of Chronos had ever had.

Jimmie and I tried to throw ourselves completely into the preparations for the Krewe of Chronos ball. I bought beautiful velvet dresses for the girls and suits for the boys. Of course, Jeanne wore a long dress because she was fourteen now, old enough to dance with the king. Watching her excitement as she got ready for the ball and seeing the way Adrienne, Robert and David's eyes sparkled, made the extra effort worth the time and emotion it consumed. Our three small children had their favorite sitter to take care of them at the ball, and we chose their seats carefully so they'd be able to see everything.

And they saw quite a magnificent king! As King Chronos, Jimmie held his shoulders back and his head up, moving regally as he waved his scepter with authority when saluting his subjects. All around me I heard, "The best king we ever had," and "He knows how to act like a king." Jimmie made people happy because he did his play-acting to the fullest that night. And he made me very proud.

On Mardi Gras day, Jimmie as King Chronos led the parade of about twenty floats and many high school bands along a winding route through the streets of Thibodaux. Tens of thousands joined in the common cry of "Throw me something, Mister!" as costumed men on floats threw thousands of colorful beads and doubloons to crowds that lined the streets. Our four children loved seeing their daddy as king. Having always been his most admiring subject, I, too, reveled in every minute. It was a grand parade.

*****

Spring went by quickly as summer and Grand Isle arrived together. Because this had always been Jimmie's favorite place to spend the long, hot, Louisiana summer days as a child, he insisted we take our children for a week's stay several times during the summer. Seashore resorts are places to forget clock watching, so Grand Isle was the ideal place for us.

Mosquitoes sometimes made us doubt the advantage of our getaway, but just seeing all four of our children have so much fun made any effort worthwhile. Each morning we made the trek to the beach and remained until the sun began to get too hot. Then back to the screened porch we went until the sun began to slip lower in the sky in the late afternoon. We again had our turn in the surf before supper each day.

Jimmie's father had given Jimmie's brother and us a yacht he had used for many years for entertaining. Now Mr. Peltier wanted us to use it for our families and friends. More a party boat than anything else, it had eight sleeping bunks and two baths. We had parties with our friends on it, but we particularly relished our family outings on the boat.

When we took everyone fishing, all the children would sit patiently with their rods, but then other interests would win out as they dashed off across the deck — except for Adrienne. Across the stern of the boat ran a little iron pipe, just the right height for her. For hours she sat on it, waiting to catch the big one. And her patience paid off as she caught her share of fish. Sand sharks were her specialty because catching one created such excitement and made her more of a celebrity than catching a speckled trout. At night, everyone fell into bed physically exhausted after the wonderful lazy times on the beach, in the fishing boat, and under the sun.

Because there were long steps to climb to our summer

home, someone always had to hold Adrienne's hand. We watched her closely at all times. As she played at the water's edge, someone sat right beside her on the beach or held her hand. I didn't ever feel she thought she was hovered over more than anyone else, and I'm sure the other children didn't resent the extra attention she received. They just accepted her as she was, not questioning. Looking back, I realize they intuitively knew she needed a little extra help.

Jimmie and I corrected Adrienne as much as we did our other children, never making them give to her what she wanted because of her problems. We worked conscientiously at disciplining her, knowing her life would be happier if she were well-behaved because no one likes a spoiled child. We had to do our part to insure she learned to get along with others, especially since she liked people so much and so enjoyed talking with anyone and everyone. Adrienne seemed independent with each thing she could do for herself, but when she needed help, she just put her hands up, knowing someone would be there. I was amused she never looked up; rather, she just put her hands up, and, of course, we always took her in our arms.

That fall, Adrienne and Robert would both be four years old. At their constant insistence, we decided to let them attend kindergarten with all their cousins near the same age. Before enrolling Adrienne, I took her over to meet her teacher and to see her school. Most of all, I wanted the teacher to see Adrienne to be sure she could handle a child with such a handicap being in the class.

Of course, some classroom activities were a problem, but Adrienne could sit down on the same kind of stool as everyone else. She was much farther advanced in handling a pencil and scissors than the other students. What worried us was the riotous free play for the last thirty to forty-minute period each day before parents picked up their children. We didn't want to take the chance of having her knocked down unintentionally. After much discussion, Jimmie and I finally decided Adrienne could adapt, and we'd let her work it out for herself. And this she did.

Sometimes Adrienne stayed in the classroom to help clean up or to write a little longer; sometimes she stood just outside the door in the play yard and talked with other girls. But waiting near the gate where the parents came to claim their children was what she liked best of all. She knew all the parents by name and enjoyed calling her friends from the play yard to tell them their parents had arrived, reminding each one to take his or her drawing of the morning. I thought it quite a feat Adrienne learned all the parent's names of those almost sixty children.

Our maid Irene spoke French. By the time Adrienne was three, she had learned to count and say her months and days in French. Anything we tried to teach her, she grasped.

Adrienne's day seemed to take on a plan. She loved music and spent a part of each day listening to records. She had her favorite TV shows, one of which was *Amos and Andy*. I don't know how she worked out her timing, but she always seemed to be in place at the exact time for a program she liked. She also found time to groom her favorite dolls with her certain brushes and combs.

Adrienne was a bit of a tease. She knew just when to look at me and laugh and when to look at me with just her eyes laughing. When we knelt to say our prayers at night and someone else was doing the reciting, she liked to giggle a little. She liked calling me back over and over at night for water or any small favor. I believe the boys coerced her to do a lot of that because they knew when she called, someone always came. She toilet trained easily. Of course, she couldn't get on a large commode by herself if the small child-size wasn't available, but she instinctively knew to ask for help if balance was required.

*****

In the late summer of 1964, the World's Fair was being

held in New York. Jimmie's sister Bernice and I decided to take Jeanne. This excursion would be a special treat for Jeanne, as well as for me. We had a spectacular time. We saw *Funny Girl* and *Hello, Dolly* in the evenings. During the day, we rented a little cart similar to a golf cart to make sure we saw everything at the fair. The three of us felt very safe going to and from Flushing Field on the subway because muggings weren't as prevalent in those days.

When Bernice, Jeanne and I were in New York, Hurricane Hilda threatened the Louisiana coast, then very quickly moved ashore in Morgan City, thirty miles west of Thibodaux. Power lines went out in Thibodaux, so telephone lines were jammed or down.

Bernice and I spent many anxious moments waiting for news. Information slowly began to trickle out of Thibodaux. We learned that practically all the Peltier family had waited the storm out at the Peltier family home except our branch. Jimmie and our three children stayed at our home eating peanut butter sandwiches. I didn't realize Jimmie could manage so well in a crisis. Fortunately, our home wasn't damaged. However, just southeast of Thibodaux in the small town of Larose, several people had been killed in tornadoes spawned by the hurricane. But by the next morning, our children hardly knew there was a blow.

Although our life at this time seemed like the normal life of our friends, it was different. Hydrocephalus was always in our thoughts. Jimmie and I could never both leave the house or be more than a telephone call away. We hadn't had any surgery in 1962 or 1963. The timing was strange. Robert arrived about two weeks after Adrienne had returned from her latest surgery at Mercy Hospital. Except for Dr. Garcia checking her periodically, she had progressed beautifully and remained well for David's arrival and during the move into our new house. Jimmie and I were afraid to put into words how well all was going.

With Adrienne fitting into our family normally, I began to

teach the children everything I could. To form the habit of them remembering each other and not taking for granted close, deep family ties, we had a big "to do" over grandparents' birthdays and anniversaries. We let the children choose the gifts, and we went on those special days to see their grandparents. I also taught them to buy their sisters and brothers presents for their birthdays.

I wanted so much for our children to be well-mannered people. Beginning in their younger years, I insisted they cover their mouths when they yawned. We tried to set examples for table manners and constantly insisted they chew with mouths closed. As this was the South, we drilled the very necessary, "Yes, Ma'am; No, Ma'am; Yes, Sir; No, Sir," until they began to incorporate those manners into their conversations. One of the most important rules, of course, was their using "Thank you." That was an absolute must.

I wanted our children to know how to behave in church as well as to show respect to God by their dressing in their best clothes for Sunday Mass. Self-discipline is one of the most important traits a person can possess, and this was one step in developing that trait.

I insisted they sit still in the pew, giving them lectures before we left for church each Sunday: "No talking; try to listen to the priest, but if your mind wanders, say the Lord's Prayer. The only reason you may speak is if you see the church on fire and you feel you have to warn everyone!"

We'd sometimes come home from church, and I'd have all three sit on an old deacon bench while I showed them how they should behave in church. Adrienne's eyes sparkled and laughed at me as I stood before them or sat beside them with my hands in my lap, looking ahead, showing them how to listen and be attentive. I had to laugh at myself when I saw how amused she was. I believe she was actually laughing at me, but with a higher intelligence than any other little girl her age. She seemed to know more about what I was trying to do than I did.

I tried to help my children develop a conscience, telling them of honor and the importance of a person giving his word, as well as the importance of being selfless and of being honest. Even if no one else knew, God would know, and they would also know when they were dishonest. I tried to teach them that as we grow older, we have to live with the mistakes we make, and we certainly don't want to look back on any dishonest deed we've done.

When my children borrowed a nickel or dime from one another, I stressed their paying it back quickly by saying, "We should all pay our bills as quickly as possible, no matter how small the amount."

When I read to them, I particularly tried to choose books with a message. One of our favorites was *The Little Engine that Could* about the train having to climb a large hill while saying, "I think I can. I think I can." I hoped they'd be like the little engine, willing to tackle hard tasks by saying, "I think I can" while giving that extra effort.

We taught them the poem, "If a task is once begun, never leave it 'til it's done. Be the labor big or small, do it well, or not at all!" I wanted the small tasks my children attempted to help them learn to complete bigger tasks later in life.

Every night I knelt down with them to say their prayers. I told them about Jesus and how He loves us. I taught them songs from my Baptist childhood, "Jesus loves me, this I know, for the Bible tells me so."

I couldn't tell them to ask Jesus for anything. I just taught them to love Him and to thank Him. The only request I could bring myself to tell them to ask was, "Please help me be good. Please let me be the person You want me to be." I'd been hurt too many times with the "no" answer; I didn't want them to have that experience.

I felt great pressure within me to teach Robert and David because I'd asked for them. I also felt pushed to teach Adrienne about values because whatever problems hydrocephalus might cause, her life would be easier with self-discipline. I was intense about teaching them values while they were young. The years would pass so quickly, and as teenagers, they wouldn't listen so readily. Because I never knew when I might be away in the hospital for long stretches, I wanted to spend quality time with them.

Jimmie and I worked equally hard at having a good time with our children. We took them crawfishing in wobbly pirogues in the back of Georgia Plantation. We spent days playing hide and seek in freshly cut hay stored in the barn over the winter months. We all admired Adrienne's patience. Once Jimmie hid her so well, no one could find her. Then he forgot where she was hidden. No matter how much all of us kept saying, "Come out. We can't find you," she remained quiet and made us find her secret spot. Seeing her laugh at all of us when she was found made the rest of us marvel at her stamina. Adrienne always played for keeps.

Jimmie and I took our children to New Orleans to ride the trolley cars on St. Charles Avenue. Jimmie would get on the trolley with them, and I'd drive down to the end of the line to pick them up. We took picnic lunches or had hot dogs at Audubon Park and Zoo. The most fun was our taking the train trip all the way around the park. Going through the tunnel excited the children, although Adrienne didn't like the sudden darkness.

We climbed through all the fiberglass animals at Storyland in City Park and rode the children's rides at Pontchartrain Beach. We carefully chose motels with children's swimming pools so they could play in the water. Of course, we took them to Walt Disney movies, the circus and the Ice Capades. Anything we thought would lead to a happier life, we tried to offer. We bought all the records children like, saving some to play for special occasions on our stereo, but allowing them to play the others on their own record player, scratches and all.

Jimmie and I always had good household help and dependable people to stay with our children at night if we wanted to go out. Hydrocephalus often interrupted our lives, but it rarely interfered. The time Jimmie and I had together was even more enhanced by hydrocephalus, so we always made outings really count. The possibility of trouble was always in the back of our minds, so we tried to make careful preparation for any eventuality, and after that, we lived as if the threat didn't exist.

In 1965, the International Oral Surgery meeting was in Copenhagen. If Jimmie and I went, we would be gone for ten days. Our help could stay with our children at our home; after all, Jimmie's mother, father, brothers and sister all lived in Thibodaux, and all the doctors knew our problem.

With every possible detail covered, Jimmie and I decided to take our first trip to Europe together. I had always heard people talk about needing a vacation. I couldn't ever identify with that need myself because my life was happy. We had the material goods to enrich the love we shared. Except for hydrocephalus, we lived a very comfortable life.

However, this trip taught me what needing a vacation meant. Travel also taught me what books, TV, or movies could never teach me. I did need a vacation, but in a different way. My mind needed that change in order to have new experiences and to grow intellectually. I needed to enrich myself as a person. New avenues of thought opened up for me. I had a desire to read more and a reason to read. Being in Europe made me want to understand the history I'd been taught. I liked walking down strange streets, floating down new rivers, and being surrounded by the European way of life. Dishes I'd always loved to cook by carefully following those complicated recipes were more exciting to eat when prepared by famous chefs in the country of their origin. I liked the feel and the excitement of a foreign country, the colors and the sounds. Being there made me feel vital, more alive.

Our first trip to Europe included visiting Madrid, so we devoted a large portion of time to the Prado Museum. I'd done my homework on the famous painters from the Spanish school and was anxious to see El Greco's elongated figures, as well as the art of Goya and Velasquez.

What I hadn't prepared for was the pictures by those artists of Jesus at various phases of His life. Up until now, I'd seen very little religious art except in books, and they were small reproductions. The spectacular scenes on huge canvases were a surprise. Each of us has our own private interpretation. I loved seeing how these great masters painted their ideas of how Jesus must have looked. My viewing the scenes of Jesus on the cross with His mother standing near by was very emotional. The artists' ability to portray the torment of heartache in the faces of those people surrounding the suffering Jesus as well as the pain and sorrow on Jesus' face captivated me. Caught up in a painting, I felt depressed seeing these suffering moments, so I'd hurry down the long halls to avoid feeling the sadness I'd been fighting back at home. Those paintings made the Lord's suffering real to me.

Being far away from home, I tried to look at my life back home more objectively. I tried to count the good and minimize the rough spots. I tried to see how I might change the bad parts or at least improve them. I felt a part of a bigger world. I felt like a dentist who does close work with his eyes all day long. The eye doctor would suggest that the dentist play golf or choose a hobby that requires looking at distances to develop that sight and relax the strain on his overworked close vision. I'd focused so long on my children, on death, and on hydrocephalus that foreign travel allowed me to use my mind to look further, to learn how big the world is, and to realize how small I'd let my world become.

Foreign travel was also having a major effect on Jimmie, but the biggest thrill for me was being with Jimmie. I loved walking the foreign streets with him and sharing the excitement of actually being in Europe.

Because Jimmie and I had made a step to expand our horizons, this pleasant trip made it easier for us to return as better parents and better people. Our time away had not seemed long to our children because there'd been no break in their routine. Rather, they seemed to appreciate us more in different ways, so Jimmie and I were happy to have made this big step to travel to Europe without our children.

*****

When our boys became American citizens, we all proudly went to the Federal Court building in New Orleans. Wearing their suits with black bow ties, Robert and David seemed very impressed with the formal ceremony. Adrienne enjoyed getting dressed up and witnessing "my boys" become citizens. We even had lunch at a fancy Italian restaurant, an experience we thought added to their education. In honor of their citizenship, a friend sent each boy a small pine tree to plant to commemorate his special day. These trees stand forty feet high today.

Sometimes the children and I planted seeds and bulbs to watch the miracle of plants growing. Once Adrienne planted a seed from a Texas grapefruit. We still enjoy that tree today because she had a part in its beginning.

*****

Christmas was more fun in 1965 because all our children were old enough to enjoy their toys and young enough to still believe in Santa. These were the fun years. We were able to give our children lots of toys because they weren't as expensive as toys for older children. I liked sitting on the steps of our sunken living room, watching all our children trying to make a path to walk among all their new possessions. Each child had his own designated spot where Santa Claus left his treasures. Christmas 1965 with all our children home was particularly grand!

Chapter Twenty-Five

Annette's Death

*J*n January 1966, the dreaded call came from Clarks – Annette was dying. Again we wanted to jump in our car and hurry to her side, but again the doctor said, "No, there is nothing you can do. Just stay right there, and we'll call you every hour!"

In the middle of that night, we knelt down and prayed, or rather, we wanted to pray. But we didn't know how to pray or what to ask for! Should we ask for Annette to get well, for a miracle? Or, should we ask God to take her quickly? Just what should we ask?

After a time, all I could pray for was that Annette not suffer. We pictured the scene far away in that dark night — our child fighting for her life. Maybe she didn't find life worth fighting for. We finally prayed, "Dear God, Thy will be done, but please don't let her have pain."

Hours stretched on. Again we knew that feeling of helplessness. Morning came; we were assured that because of the coma, Annette wasn't aware of anything and her death was imminent, but this struggle of her body dying could take time. Nurses were beside her every minute, and doctors were readily available. Nothing more could be done.

Again Jimmie and I had to wait.

Annette had been away for five years. She hadn't been

aware of the world around her since she was eighteen months old. Now, at nine years of age, she was dying. I felt sorrow for her wasted life and the pain she suffered. Always there was the unanswered question, "Why? Why was Annette born like this?"

I felt painfully deprived of my baby girl. I thought of how much I'd have loved rearing that beautiful little blonde girl. Life seemed unfair when an innocent little baby suffered so terrible a condition. All the memories of Jim came flooding back, of Benita Ann, of all the heartaches we'd experienced during those years that seemed like an eternity.

Then I felt deep sorrow because I didn't know what lay ahead for Adrienne, who was to be six in March. She had been well since 1961. We'd been spared for a time from the trauma the hydrocephalic treatments demanded. But now all the horrors came back, and the knowledge that more were coming haunted me. No one else, not even our parents, could begin to understand the complexity of the sorrow Jimmie and I shared only with one another.

Around three o'clock, the final call came that Annette had passed away. I grieved because I felt I never really knew Annette. Because she was the sickest of our four, it was difficult to believe she'd outlived Benita Ann. She'd been number four, born into a home where two other children had hydrocephalus and a healthy one-year-old was just beginning to walk. I held her, rocked her, fed her, and bathed her, but I didn't seem to have as much extra time to devote to her as I had for all my others. When each of our other three children were infants, I'd had more time. Taking care of four children meant each one couldn't have as much of my attention as I wanted to give. Even when Annette was in the hospital, she had to share that experience with a sister. I knew I'd done everything I could for Annette, but I regretted and blamed myself for not being able to give more of me to Annette.

I dreaded yet another funeral. No matter how many one lives through, nothing is so final and depressing as the profound finality of burying one of your dead. I knew I should accept Annette's death as a blessing for her because this day she'd be with God. She'd entered into what we all eventually want. I should have felt fortunate to have another angel in Heaven, but I had trouble trying to think positively.

I didn't want to hear all the pretty speeches from well-meaning friends again or make them go through another funeral. So we tried to keep Annette's death quiet, make no announcements, and have the funeral very quickly. But in Thibodaux, there is no way to keep anything so newsworthy quiet.

I must admit that when I saw our friends arrive, I felt differently. I guess I'd wanted to run away from the discomfort our sorrow and their duty to come and be consoling was imposing on our friends. I was surprised when their coming did console me. Their presence, their just being there, made me understand I couldn't remove myself from the world and have my unhappy thoughts alone. Their presence made me realize how important all of us are to each other, how we need others in our sorrow even as we know they don't fully experience the depths of our loss.

I was going through a strange time. Because I was never alone, it was hard to think. People were around me, and I couldn't cry. The nuns and people who came from Clarks did make me feel better because someone who knew Annette was with me. They could tell us about her and remind us again how marvelous a place the home had been for her to finish those unknowing years.

I was amazed at the big crowds who came to Annette's funeral Mass on such short notice. The church filled again for a child no one knew. But this time I felt to be present for Annette's funeral Mass was a special treat because God was being given another saint in Heaven. Annette's was a different kind of funeral, one in which our child was released from her pain to live a glorious life with God.

Then something else happened; Jimmie's family invited

all the nuns over to their house after the funeral. Jimmie and I were all alone at home with our heavy hearts, having lost three out of our four with hydrocephalus.

This time Jimmie and I suffered individually. Of course, we thought of each other, but it was as if we had to try to pull our thinking back together individually to again accept our life. Since we'd known Annette so little, this time Jimmie and I had a chance to feel sorry for ourselves, and we didn't feel this seemed selfish at all.

*****

On March 4, 1966, Adrienne was six years old. Because her birthday was near Easter, we always had an Easter party with individual Easter egg cakes from Gambino's Bakery in New Orleans and an Easter egg hunt. Each guest received a basket to gather his eggs, played "Pin the Tail on the Donkey," guessed the correct number of beans in a jar, and played any kind of game that had lots of the guests winning prizes. A lady in town came to perform in her clown outfit, and the children liked that.

I tried to give each of my children the best birthday party possible, but Adrienne's meant something special because she had lived happily for yet another year. This particular year was a milestone because she'd begin school in September.

Adrienne had straight blonde hair she loved to brush and groom. Hairdressers suggested she wear bangs over her larger forehead, but she liked a barrette like her friends, so I didn't fight her ideas. If she wanted a barrette, fine! She was all female; she liked clothes, shoes, and hair styling from the beginning. We wanted her to wear sturdy supportive shoes, but she liked to wear my shoes. She wore a pair of black ballet-type slippers around the house, the back of which stuck out a full three inches past her heels. She liked her fancy nightgowns and pretty long robes. She felt pretty; she was pretty; and I told her so.

From the very first time I read aloud to Adrienne, she liked books. In fact, she memorized books at around age two and could actually sit beside her brothers with her books and read aloud. As she repeated the words, she even turned the page at the correct moment. Adrienne handled a pencil beautifully and learned to print quickly.

She was a busybody, always keeping up with what everyone was doing. I had to watch that she didn't boss "my boys." TV occupied a large part of her spare time, and she introduced to our family the saying, "The TV is mine, heard it or not, understood it or not!"

When she had to vacate her spot in front of the TV, that was the announcement she made, assuming everyone was within earshot. Of course, she rarely got arguments from the boys, Jeanne, or me.

The stereo also claimed time in her life. "Ode to Billy Joe," "Love is Blue," and "See the Tree How Big It's Grown" by Bobby Goldsboro were among her favorites; however, I didn't understand why she liked these sad songs.

People all over town knew Adrienne from nursery school. She met people there I didn't even know. Learning people's names came naturally to her, and at her station at the gate, she talked to all the parents when they came to claim their children. When we went to the dime stores or grocery stores together, everyone said to her, "Hello, Adrienne," and she would reply using their names, "Hello, Mrs. So-and-so." She seemed to know everyone everywhere we went. My other children and I found ourselves looking at those people in amazement, and then the person would smile and nod to the rest of us.

Kindergarten lasted all day at St. Joseph School. Even though Robert was the same age as Adrienne, we chose to put them in separate classes so they wouldn't rival each other. Even at school, Adrienne was a busybody, knew everyone's name, and loved to recite in front of the class.

Adrienne loved every subject at school. Any challenge in numbers or words made her light up. Religion class was of special interest to her. I began to hear her ask people, "Are you going up or down?"

At first, I didn't understand what she meant, but she explained this meant Heaven or Hell. Each one of us had to decide and work toward a goal. Heaven was her goal. I suppose she was just checking to see what everyone else planned to do.

Adrienne rode the bus to kindergarten like everyone else in our neighborhood. Since we were one of the first bus stops, she always had a seat. The bus driver showed extra patience in making sure she had plenty of time to ascend and descend the steps. She had such a winning smile I believe he learned to love her, too.

To watch Adrienne leave on the bus in the morning was hard. Someone was always available and could be reached in a second if there were any need for me, but I worried so about her falling. I hired help that could drive in case they were needed to get her from school. I don't think the boys and Jeanne were aware of how much we kept ourselves so available for Adrienne. Of course, we were also there for them, but we built our plans around Adrienne because this had to be done.

The highlight of my day was when my children would return from school. The boys would come running out of the bus. Not too far behind was Adrienne running through the deep rye grass across our front yard with papers in her hand. She didn't seem to notice that she always brought up the rear, but my heart broke as I stood there watching. Maybe I shouldn't have tried so hard to integrate her life with that of other children so she wouldn't feel different, but I did, and I have no regrets.

*****

Each hour of each day, I appreciated how fortunate we were to be living normal lives. I was beginning, just beginning, to relax my interior thoughts and to stop waiting for bad news. Suddenly, Adrienne began to have headaches. At first, these didn't occur too often or for very long periods. As much as we tried to hope the headaches were caused by something else, we knew there must be problems with the shunt, so we drove to New Orleans to see Dr. Garcia.

We could feel that tubing beneath the skin behind Adrienne's right ear as it came out of her skull before going back into her body on its way to her heart. Dr. Garcia had to force through any sediment that might be slowing the fluid flowing through the tube to her heart.

He used a special stripping procedure to assist the draining process. Adrienne would lie on her left side as Vaseline or a greasy cream would be applied to the area. With the thumb of his left hand, Dr. Garcia would press down very firmly on the end of the tube nearest her skull. He placed his right thumb next to his left thumb and applied pressure for two or three inches down the tubing with the right thumb.

Dr. Garcia repeated this stripping two or three times with his right thumb before he released the pressure with his left thumb. A valve in the shunt prevented the fluid from flowing back into Adrienne's head. So the pressure opened this valve and helped the excess spinal fluid flow into the chamber of Adrienne's heart, relieving the pressure inside her head causing her headache.

At first, only Dr. Garcia would perform this procedure. But after Jimmie and I made several visits to the emergency room in New Orleans, he taught us how to give Adrienne relief. No matter how firm the person's hands were that did the stripping, Adrienne seemed to feel no discomfort.

Because Jimmie and I so wanted to make Adrienne's life all right and free from hydrocephalus, our name for this stripping process evolved to "make it all right." If Adrienne didn't feel well, either of us would ask, "Do you want me to make it all right?"

We were to hear that phrase morning, noon, and night many, many times. What a boon to our life this seemed to be. On request, we could strip the tubing and turn Adrienne's dull look of not feeling well into her immediately jumping up feeling great. Now Jimmie and I never left town at the same time because someone had to be available on short notice to "make it all right."

Adrienne continued to go to school. If she needed help, her teacher had the school secretary contact us. Within minutes, we could reach her, and in a small room off the principal's office, we'd perform this procedure. Then back to class Adrienne would go. I don't know what sort of discomfort she felt. I didn't want to ask. But whatever she felt, she did ask for help quickly. As time went on, we taught our household help how to "make it all right." The procedure became so routine that we had fewer anxieties and only felt we needed to be near when we were needed.

Adrienne excelled in first grade. Her hours in class passed all too quickly because she liked reading, writing and arithmetic, always wanting more. She had to overcome her desire to talk to her neighbors in class, but at recess time, she had children all around her as she talked with them. Even with her peers, Adrienne showed a deep interest in each as a person, always knowing their names and remembering their interests. The boys liked her, also. There was always a boyfriend.

I often felt sorry for Adrienne's teacher, but she accepted the problem, became a good friend of Adrienne's, and enjoyed seeing her gobble up any new knowledge. There seemed to be no apprehension on the part of anyone at the school, least of all Adrienne. She never worried that there might be no one there to "make it all right." She just knew we would be there. She never questioned this new feeling of hers. But we found ourselves wondering, wondering what was going on inside her little body.

Adrienne looked so adorable in the brown skirt and blouse that was her school uniform. When the Teeny Tiny football game time came, she marched on the football field with a red skirt, white blouse and a very special made, over-sized beanie hat, looking like every other little girl.

The Teeny Tiny football game had been a tradition for

thirty years. Jimmie had been captain of the team in 1939. The fourth, fifth, and sixth grade boys made up the team while all the other students participated in the auxiliary entertainment. This, of course, made every parent want to attend, making this football game the best money-making event the Mother's Club ever had.

Every parent's face was aglow as their children did their small part to make this event successful. No parent in the stands could have felt the love and joy Jimmie and I did when we watched Adrienne. She sat with her group. There was never any hanging on to us or whining. Adrienne happily charged at life, always wanting it all. She had no insecure feelings. Even sitting so far away from us in the stands, she knew that by simply asking, we could be had. She smiled and cheered and, as usual, talked during the entire game. That night we put to bed a tired little girl who had fit in perfectly with her peers.

When Adrienne went to visit friends, she always knew all she had to do was ask the mother to call us and help would be on the way. She wasn't frightened of anything. She had her life under control. In reality, she had the five of us under control, also!

One morning as Jimmie drove past Adrienne's school, he noticed a class of small ones walking single file to the playground. There was Adrienne at the head of the line, holding hands and chattering with the teacher. Suddenly, Adrienne jumped out in front of the line, raised one arm, and halted the group. She walked back to a little boy who'd apparently been misbehaving. Jimmie could see Adrienne giving the little boy a stern lecture, shaking her finger at him. Then he saw the little boy's head bow dejectedly as Adrienne marched back to the front, grasped the teacher's hand, and waved the column forward. We often wondered what that teacher thought. Jimmie sat and watched in stunned silence. Adrienne was a born leader.

One day, I turned to Adrienne as she sat beside me on the front seat of the car and gave me a big over done smile. I realized then she must have been imitating me. Each time I looked at her, I'd give a big smile of happiness, so I guess she thought she'd return it. When I realized her smile was a little much, I tried after that not to grin so enthusiastically every time I looked at her.

Adrienne had many things worked out in her mind. One day while riding home from town on one of the long, joy-filled drives living in the country afforded me, Adrienne was standing on the floor in the back, holding on to the back of the front seat. Robert and David were having a conversation about the difference between boys and girls. With a toss of her head, she very matter-of-factly said, "Everyone knows that boys have short hair, and girls have long hair." In 1966, the effect of the Beatles hadn't yet been felt in Thibodaux.

*****

First grade hadn't dealt so kindly with Robert. That year, classes were woefully overcrowded. He had an inexperienced teacher who didn't know how to deal with over-exuberant boys, Robert included. She separated the boys from the rest of the class and taught first grade to the others. As a result, Robert made good grades, but he didn't learn how to read. Even though Robert was promoted to second grade, he wasn't prepared.

Jimmie and I spent many hours deliberating about what to do. A very close friend who'd taught first grade for thirty years came to visit. After hearing Robert read, she immediately said, "He should have the opportunity to repeat the first grade."

Having a December birthday, Robert was actually eleven months younger than some of his classmates. That would make him feel more comfortable repeating the first grade. So Jimmie and I decided to make a decision based on our friend's recommendation.

We transferred Robert from parochial school to public school, giving him a new environment. He wouldn't see his classmates go on to the second grade, and his new first grade teacher, who had a PhD, said she'd like the challenge of helping him.

Adrienne depended on Robert to help her with her bus rides and other things. With Robert in another school, she'd miss his help. So we decided she, too, should transfer to public school if the principal and teachers would accept her. I took Adrienne to meet all the new teachers and the school secretary. Her distinct way of speaking seemed to enchant all of them. Of course, they'd be happy to enroll her.

A few days before the opening day of school, I took Adrienne to her second grade teacher's home so they could get to know each other. Adrienne looked very pretty in her new dress as she sat properly in a straight back chair for an interview. After she and the teacher spoke a while, Adrienne said, "I'll have to be first in line when the class goes to lunch."

Of course, the teacher hastened to explain how others also needed an opportunity to be first. Adrienne understood the explanation about sharing, but what we didn't know was she was right. She needed someone to hold her hand to keep her going at a certain speed. Being in a hurry, the other children walked too rapidly for her. If she were placed in the middle of the line, there'd be a big gap between her and the person ahead of her. So one day after school had been in session for a while, Adrienne came home saying, "Mrs. Webre realized I'd have to walk along with her at the front of the line!"

For a few years Adrienne had watched Jeanne take piano lessons. She couldn't wait to be in second grade so she could begin to play the piano. The piano teacher's house was only half a mile from our house, so Adrienne would get off the bus there. The bus driver would help her off the bus, walk across the street with her, and Mrs. Marshall, the teacher, would wait for Adrienne on the front porch. I'd pick her up thirty minutes later.

I always felt guilty about these arrangements. I wanted to pick Adrienne up at school, drive her to her lessons, and wait for her, but we were trying to rear her for her future. And Adrienne wanted to do it that way because the other students were doing it that way.

During the summer before she entered second grade, Adrienne developed a strange symptom. She would become very frigid and shake for a short time. Her teeth would even chatter. We'd give her a hot pad to hold and cover her with warm blankets. There seemed to be no explanation for this new symptom. Dr. Garcia didn't offer any reason nor recommend any treatment.

Adrienne didn't seem upset by this at all. The minute she felt cold, she told someone, and we sat with her as she held the hot pad. There was a room near the principal's office with a small bed where she was able to lie down. Jimmie and I were always called, and one of us always went to sit with her. As soon as she stopped shaking, she got right up to hurry back to class. This problem had no relationship with the shunt needing to be stripped. There was no definite pattern; it didn't happen every day or every week; however, it might even happen two or three times in one day. Adrienne never complained about this new inconvenience. She was made of pure determination. There were no tears. She took the shakes in stride just as she did everything else.

Chapter Twenty-Six

Adrienne Is Not Well

$\mathcal{I}$ trained my servants to know exactly what to do for Adrienne and pushed myself to participate in the social life of Thibodaux in spite of, or maybe because of, our worries with hydrocephalus. In order to be a decent mate to my husband, it was necessary I have other interests so our life together wouldn't only be talk of sick children. I wasn't going to retreat into a shell because of the perplexities we had.

Two years had passed since our last trip to Europe, a trip that had been rewarding to both Jimmie and me. We decided this would be a good time and a safe time to leave for two weeks, so we carefully planned our trip to Paris and England.

We took Adrienne to the local pediatrician, who said there was no reason why we shouldn't be able to go. Since we had no way of knowing Adrienne's future, he thought it wise we get away together for a while and insisted we go. He'd watch Adrienne closely, and a phone call to Europe would be simple enough if we were needed. Adrienne had been having it "made all right" for almost one and a half years; the shakes hadn't made any noticeable change in her health; and people were there who could care for her.

Every minute plan possible was made so our household

with our four children could function smoothly. Our four children were happily settled in school. Nothing more we could do would add to their comfort, happiness and security, so we departed for Paris in October.

After only three days in Paris, Jimmie and I received a call from our family pediatrician friend, Dr. Ernest Hansen. Before he could say anything, we knew the news wasn't good. In my nervousness, I felt more alert than ever, sitting there while Jimmie took the call and seeing every detail in our lovely room at the Plaza Athenee as I never had before. The beautiful linen on the beds, the thick-quilted comforters, and the sweeping elegance of the drapes stood out so vividly. When terrible news suddenly plunders our mind, I wonder if our mind tends to reject the bad news by noticing more acutely the world around us.

Dr. Hansen said, "Adrienne is in heart failure. Everything is being done for her. Both her grandmothers and Dottie Toups, your cousin who's a registered nurse, are with her. We thought you'd want to know. Adrienne is happy and comfortable, and no one will do anything until you get home, but you should leave now!"

Jimmie and I just looked at each other as he told me, "Don't think about it. There will be plenty of time to think when we get home. Just try to get things together to pack, and I'll call the travel agent here in Paris to get us out of here."

We found out what having an expert travel agent means. Mr. André Chalufor said, "I'm sorry about the bad news, Dr. Peltier. Pack your bags; don't check out; just meet me in twenty minutes with your luggage in front of the hotel."

Jimmie and I moved as if we were directed by a computer. Mr. Chalufor was exact in his timing. On the way to the airport, he said, "There are always two seats saved on airplanes in first class until the last minute for V.I.P.'s. I've secured these seats for you."

I tried to pray as we drove through the streets of Paris that beautiful fall day as my mind was again seeking the beauty around me. The autumn leaves were just turning; people were rushing down the Champs Elyseé as always. People dining at the sidewalk cafés looked so happy. When we met the traffic jam around the Arc de Triomphe, I could see into every car—people smiling and in love. I felt so removed from them because I was in another world from theirs. I was in a world all my own with generous portions of fear and sorrow.

Mr. Chalufor accompanied us to check our luggage, came with us through security, and remained with us until our flight was announced. He didn't say much. He was just there, such a comfort to us both. This man must have suffered a great tragedy in his life to take the time from his busy day to sit with perfect strangers. The surprise of having his kindness and his concern directed toward us felt as if he represented mankind, and that mankind wanted to say to me, "No matter how bad the times are, we other human beings are here and care although we can do nothing to ease your burden."

When I shook Mr. Chalufor's hand and tried to look deep into his eyes, I hope he knew his kindly efforts warranted more than the "Thank you" I was able to smile and say.

Our flight home made no memories; instead, it was a time spent in confused numbness. I tried to exact from Jimmie's knowledge what heart failure meant. Even my Rock of Gibraltar didn't know what this new development meant. He just knew it wasn't good and said, "Wait. You'll have enough time to think about it later."

When we reached home, there were my mother, Jimmie's mother, Dottie Toups, and Grace and Bernice, my two sisters-in-law. They had taken Adrienne to a cardiologist in Baton Rouge. I didn't even understand his diagnosis. As I did try to listen and grasp what had been done for her, Jimmie and I were more interested in getting Adrienne to New Orleans to Dr. Garcia.

Even with heart failure, Adrienne was very much in charge of everything. She didn't seem frightened by all this new attention. She was happy to see us and seemed as alert as always, but she was unable to walk or exert any effort. I had the same strength I had been blessed with when Jim needed me as his legs, so I could pick Adrienne up and carry her distances with no problem.

Jimmie and I explained it was necessary for her to go to New Orleans to see Dr. Garcia, and that suited her fine. She just wanted a pair of penny loafers like the ones her friends wore. Shifting my priorities to penny loafers was hard as I said, "I'll manage some way some how to find some small enough for you. When we get to New Orleans, I'll get on the phone and call everywhere until I find some!"

On October 6, 1967, we began nine months that would demand more of Jimmie and me than I thought two people capable of enduring while they still try to be normal, happy people after the siege is over.

Most of the ensuing events remain a little hazy in my mind because I wanted it that way. All the medical procedures that had to be done were out of my control. I couldn't contribute to their success or failure. However, during my child's waking hours, as well as during her sleeping hours, I could play a giant part to try to keep Adrienne happy, entertained, and comfortable to the very best of my ability. That was to be my whole purpose in life.

Because we'd known many of this medical group for thirteen years, Jimmie gave the nursing staff specific instructions, "We have a very sick little girl here with an unknown future. We're going to make her stay as comfortable as possible. Please don't talk about a shot in front of her. If a shot is to be given, come with the shot, needle out of sight, tell her, and give it quickly. Don't prolong her anxiety. She's brave. For anything you have to do that's going to be uncomfortable for her, get all of your equipment together, come in, and do the blood test or whatever without any pre-discussion to cause her any anxiety. Then get all your things together, and get out."

Adrienne was assigned to Room 514. Our other three

children each had a turn using this room in the past. After Adrienne's admission into the hospital, Jimmie and I began the ritual we must have been through one hundred times — settling into a hospital room. The laboratory technician came to take a blood sample. The nurse brought in a small container for a urine specimen. The television man came to ask if we wanted to rent a television set. The rental company offered the service of renting a rollaway bed for the mother staying with the patient.

I'd been through all of these steps so many times before. Each step made me cringe because I was panicky, not knowing the implication this admission would have on all of us. No admission had ever resulted in happiness for us.

My head was swimming with the memories of all the previous times spent in the many hospital rooms with our four children suffering, each at different ages and different stages. Their faces always gazed up from the white sheets, their eyes showing trust and love as they looked at Jimmie and me. In a way, I always felt I'd betrayed that trust because they suffered from hydrocephalus. I reminded myself we had no other choice. We had to accept the surgeries medical science offered from 1954 to 1967. The situation demanded we acquiesce to what the best doctors could recommend to help our four precious children.

I tried to dress the best I could, keep my face in repair, and look confidently happy. The keep-smiling part wasn't so hard because I loved being near Adrienne. She made me feel good. She had many interests and kept me busy handing her this item or reading her that book. But this time penny loafers is what she wanted. She didn't seem to forget anything.

After making many calls, I finally found a pair at J.C. Penny's. I drew a map showing her where J.C. Penny was located in relation to the hospital. Then I gave her my watch as I told her I'd be back with the loafers when the big hand reached a certain number. I insisted she'd have to read or entertain herself for that length of time.

After a lot of rushing, I was able to buy the shoes and get back to Adrienne on time. She wore the loafers in her bed during her waking hours. From then on, I was able to get a sandwich or other food with my watch as a ransom. Adrienne tried to be patient, but she wanted me with her every minute.

Tests were run, and without the doctors telling me, I could see they were hesitant to tamper with the shunt. It was draining, and her hydrocephalus was arrested. But her heart was rejecting the presence of a foreign body, the tubing going into the chamber of her heart. Her heart failure became worse.

After two weeks of careful planning, Dr. Garcia and a cardiologist took Adrienne to surgery and removed the tubing going into her heart. A new tubing was attached to her shunt and brought down into the peritoneal cavity, allowing the spinal fluid to drain into her stomach instead of her heart. The tubing removed from Adrienne's heart was then cultured to check for infection. Two weeks later, the culture revealed Adrienne had had bacterial endocarditis, an inflammation of the lining around her heart. I believe Dr. Garcia had known this long ago but wasn't inclined to replace her tubing until now.

Before Adrienne's operation, Jimmie was able to get full cooperation from the operating room staff, so we decided not to tell Adrienne she was having surgery. Rather, we introduced her to the anesthetist. Liking people as much as she did, Adrienne was anxious to go into their part of the hospital for a visit. Jimmie was allowed to go into the operating room with her and make her laugh as he showed her different pieces of equipment and chatted with the hospital staff. They were able to get her to slip off to sleep without her being aware of what was happening. Because I'd nursed hydrocephalic patients for what now amounted to thirteen years, Dr. Garcia didn't send Adrienne to the recovery room as is the case with every other surgical patient. Instead, he allowed her to be brought to her room so that when she opened her eyes, I was standing there. She never seemed to be concerned about bandages, and for some reason, never asked why they were there.

For a time, she felt bad and lay still. Soon she was able to sit up and get busy again, charged at getting the most out of every day. To treat heart failure, the drug digitalis is used. Those injections can be painful. Adrienne was a real trooper about getting injections, but a few seconds after getting the digitalis injection, she'd begin to scream. There must have been a terrible burning sensation to cause such pain and make her cry as she did for up to twenty minutes sometimes.

Little could I do to give her comfort until the pain was gone. I just wanted to pick her up and leave the hospital, never to return – anything to prevent her from receiving those painful shots. But I was completely at the mercy of the medical staff. I didn't know what to do for her, but there were times I felt they didn't know either.

I got so mad at God that I pictured myself looking up and saying, "I hope You're happy. How could seeing a child suffer be pleasing to You?"

Then I'd feel ashamed... but, nevertheless, this thought persisted. Jimmie and I never discussed Adrienne's illness in her presence. Doctors seemed careful not to say too much in her room. She seemed to trust us and do whatever we said. I certainly never sat down and explained anything to her because there seemed no need. Why frighten a child when she didn't seem concerned about what was happening?

I gave myself completely to Adrienne. Sometimes I felt as if I were an extension of her. We were like one. I felt she drew strength from me. To have one's body so very ill is horrible. To look up from a hospital bed into someone else's eyes and know that person has no feeling for you would be even more horrible. But when a patient has someone caring for her who loves her more than life itself, surely the ravages of the illness and the mental anguish must be easier to bear. Adrienne and I were like two people suspended in time — each dedicated to making the other person's hour a joy. She worked at loving and giving of herself to me as I did to her. I wished I could have suffered and had the illness instead of her.

When Adrienne felt well, it was obvious. Between shots, Adrienne and I had fun. Some of the happiest hours of my life were spent in her room. During one of those good days, I called a priest to see if we could get a Bishop to confirm her. She'd never made her First Communion either. I wasn't going to leave any sacrament undone in her life I could manage to get administered, so Bishop Abel Caillouet, who was originally from Thibodaux, came to the hospital to give Adrienne First Communion as well as to confirm her.

I wanted so much to ask her to pray to get well while receiving these two great sacraments, but I didn't want her to be hurt by God as I'd been. I'd always loved and believed the promise of Jesus, "Everything you ask my Father in my name will be given to you." But I'd learned long ago that the sentence, "Thy will be done," took precedence over the other request.

I'd worked at teaching Adrienne to love God and tried to reassure her He loved her. But I didn't want her to know that just a word from Him could cure her. I'd have been hurt more knowing He had turned her down. One could say I was protecting myself and saw no reason for us both to be hurt by Him more deeply.

The moments Adrienne received Communion and Confirmation were powerful moments. Knowing God was here in the room with us, more present than ever, all I could do was stand by and bow my head. In that one instant, He could have cured her, but that wasn't His choice.

As these momentous happenings were taking place, I often thought, *Something is going on that is much bigger than I, but I feel nothing. I just know it's happening.*

I just wish I could have understood, even partially understood, God's plan because I believe He has one. What good could come from having our little girl suffer? That question was always with me during those long hours.

As I followed the Bishop out into the hall, I offered to pay him for coming, but he shook his head. He must have felt as

I did, that the sacraments he had just administered provided him with a rare privilege to give them to one of God's angels. Adrienne was lovely in a striking way, and I realized others besides me thought of her as one of God's angels, too.

Now Adrienne had received her first Communion, the priest who brought daily Communion to hospital patients brought Communion to us both after Mass every morning. Each day we could hear the tinkling of the bell as the priest got off the elevator and made his way down the hospital corridor. I could also see Adrienne's eyes dancing with mischief. Maybe she was amused by the reverence or maybe it was her sheer joy at receiving Jesus. She couldn't wait until she could walk down the aisle at St. Joseph Church to receive Communion. I must confess that each morning when we received the sacrament, I still begged Jesus to cure Adrienne.

If only Adrienne could have been spared her pain. Just the peculiar life she had to lead away from school and friends she loved was suffering enough. The bodily pain seemed so unnecessary.

I got through those seizures of pain by sheer discipline. The minute Adrienne's pain stopped and her eyes clearly sought me out, I put the unpleasant last minutes out of my mind completely and concentrated on the present ones. I didn't spend time dreading the pain again or worrying about whatever else might happen. When that minute came, I'd have plenty of time for that desperate feeling I'd come to know. I literally took one hour at a time, blocking out the bad from my memory. There was never time in those days to reflect and remember... no roses to smell along the way.

*****

Adrienne used to grade papers for her second-grade teacher. One day she announced, "I'm ready to grade papers,"

I rushed to the telephone to call Jimmie so he could bring papers to grade that night. Adrienne couldn't wait to correct the tests. After working for a while, she said very matter-of-factly,

"Well, Mack has certainly improved since the beginning of the year. He's much neater and forms his letters more clearly."

This was three months after school had started! I was impressed with that being said by a seven-year-old. Adrienne was very advanced.

Other times, she'd say, "I'm lonesome for a book. Could you get one for me?"

Again a phone call, and since everyone was devoted to making Adrienne happy, again the book would quickly arrive.

Through the years, Jimmie was always turning up with a new, endearing nickname for her. "Miss Lizzie" was one of my favorites. About this time, Adrienne didn't want me out of her sight in the hospital and was constantly saying, "Mama, Mama."

Jimmie began to call her "Poupee-qui-dit, Mama," the doll that says Mama. She loved the name and would say it over and over.

Although Jimmie and I were closer than ever, we each had a pattern to follow. He was at home with our other three children, trying to make them happy and help them lead a normal life. I had to be with Adrienne in the hospital. It wasn't in any sense of the word normal family living.

Jimmie and I made frequent telephone calls to each other. He knew all that went on in Adrienne's hospital room every day, came at least every other night, and kept me informed about what was taking place at home. I felt sorry he had to make that long trip back and forth to New Orleans alone because there was too much time for him to think about Adrienne.

The nurses waived the visiting rules on the doctor's orders, allowing Jeanne, Robert, and David to come visit when Adrienne was having a good day. We wanted them to see her in hospital surroundings in order to prevent them from picturing something horrible; however, we didn't share our worries with them. We didn't feel they should know each time Adrienne had infusions or that frequent injections were prescribed. We arranged their visits so she could also enjoy her brothers and sister.

Several times she'd say, "You know, Mama, I'm lonesome for Jeanne."

Of course, we rushed Jeanne in whenever she talked like that. We also let her talk on the telephone as often as possible. Adrienne had an admiring audience all over the hospital who visited often; however, I guarded her, checked all her medicine carefully, and kept people out when she dozed off to sleep.

Adrienne's headaches started again. This new peritoneal shunt didn't have a tubing that could be stripped to allow it to drain better. A few hours after the doctors realized the shunt wasn't draining properly, she was taken to surgery to determine why she was having this problem.

Only ten days after the removal of her cardiac shunt tubing, the new peritoneal shunt needed adjustment. On October 27, 1969, the cervical portion of Adrienne's ventriculo-peritoneal shunt needed to be revised.

Again, Jimmie and I both went down to surgery with her. Jimmie was allowed into the operating room until she received the anesthetic. I was thankful she didn't have to go to the recovery room; instead, she came back to me in her hospital room to awaken.

Adrienne was the bravest little sport, never a complaint unless she was writhing in pain. If there were any way she could feel well, she did. It was almost like mind over matter. We were blessed she was a happy person and looked at the bright side of everything.

This time her revised shunt did work. Although she couldn't walk around because she was too weak and still affected by her heart failure, she could be carried everywhere. With big smiles, we all went back to Thibodaux on November 4. Jeanne, Robert and David accepted us back into their lives as though we hadn't been away.

*****

Adrienne looked beautiful to me, forever smiling and

happy. Again she organized her day. By now, she'd learned how to embroider. She spent time watching TV, some time sewing, a lot of time reading, and a lot of time listening to music. She played cards and could shuffle those cards perfectly. She always found time to groom her dolls, brushing their hair and changing their clothes. She had a little play world all her own on her counterpane, and she brightened everybody's life.

One day when Adrienne and I were alone, I remembered how shaken I'd been after Jim died when I realized I had trouble picturing his face. No matter how hard I tried, his face seemed to elude me.

With that loss gnawing at me, I lay down by Adrienne as she lay in my bed and watched television. I rubbed her feet. Then I closed my eyes, trying to commit her feet to memory. I rubbed her legs with lotion and did the same, trying to make an indelible print on my mind so I'd never forget. I did this with her little hands and fingers, her wrists and elbows, and her little neck and face. I studied each detail—her forehead with small scars where she'd fallen many times and bumped her head because it was so heavy, the part in her hair, her cowlick, her ears, and the feel of her hair.

I loved Adrienne so much I was trying to insure I'd never forget any detail of her body should I ever need to draw on my memory someday. Adrienne was unaware of what I was doing because I always put lotion on her skin to keep it smooth and healthy.

Jimmie and I had no problems carrying her everywhere in our arms. Although she'd lost some weight, she was seven-and-a-half years old and still rather heavy. She still had enough strength to sit upright, but her heart was weak, and the doctors felt she shouldn't ever exert herself. I happily spent time taking her everywhere.

Amos and Andy was her favorite TV show. One day when the announcement was made the show would be cancelled in a few weeks, she wrote the network asking them to keep it. I constantly marveled at her intelligence and interest in life.

We tried to cook food she liked and did our best to keep her well nourished. Nothing was too much trouble. Jimmie surprised her with a TV for the kitchen so we could distract her mind, hoping she'd eat more.

Jimmie also surprised me with a gift. He jokingly said that since we didn't have to pay a nurse to take care of Adrienne, he bought me a present with my fee for being her nurse… a pair of sapphire and diamond earrings in the shape of a camellia. I was so touched he thought of me when he was having to struggle to accept his daily sufferings.

Jimmie and I also decided to build a beach house on Grand Isle near the edge of the Gulf of Mexico. It would be a good place for Adrienne to recuperate and get her strength back. The beach house was on pilings to protect it from hurricanes and had many windows to create a cross draft for the Gulf breeze. A sundeck on the beach side of the house allowed Adrienne to see the water, and steps leading down from the sundeck to the sand allowed us to take her to be near the surf. All of us were excited about our beach house.

*****

Unfortunately, Adrienne's headaches and discomfort returned, obviously indicating her shunt had ceased draining. We rushed back to New Orleans on December 14, this time having no time to pack luggage. We just picked Adrienne up and left.

Dr. Garcia checked her as the anesthetist and all the operating room staff were summoned. The time seemed to last forever before Adrienne was prepped and taken to surgery as quickly as the evening schedule allowed. After she'd been taken from her hospital room, Jimmie said, "Nothing can happen for an hour. Let's go check into a motel and eat." Not have dinner. *Eat.* We always were hungrier when times were bad.

When we arrived at the motel, the man on duty required us to pay in advance since we had no luggage. Jimmie and I just looked at each other and laughed. Why let anything excite us when our baby was lying on the operating table a few blocks down the street?

So Jimmie and I went back to our favorite steakhouse where we'd eaten great juicy steaks all these years we'd spent at Mercy Hospital. We'd never been out of the hospital before when surgery was in progress, but Adrienne's procedure would last eight or nine hours. We knew the first two hours couldn't possibly demand our being there, and at least two hours would be needed to get her to sleep and to prepare and position her for surgery.

Through all our children's surgeries, this was the first time Jimmie and I thought of ourselves. We both were trying to save a little stretch of time to gain some composure, time just for us. In that little family-type New Orleans restaurant, we sat across from each other in a dimly lit booth with the curtain drawn, our hands touching as we talked. I almost felt as though we were in a bubble, isolated from the world. We wanted normal things like a drink and supper. We hoped we'd leave that bubble and enter whatever this new surgery would mean to Adrienne's life and ours.

When supper was over, Jimmie and I went back to the hospital to resume our vigil, which lasted all night. At dawn, Adrienne was wheeled back into Room 504 with the statement, "We did what we set out to do," ringing in our ears. Dr. Garcia had revised her peritoneal shunt. Adrienne seemed to be recovering well from surgery. She was her old self, laughing as much as possible.

Dr. Garcia ordered meals to be sent to her three times a day. I fed her what she could eat and ate the rest. I didn't leave her for a moment since there was no one but me to stay. Adrienne still lived up to her name, "Poupee qui dit, Mamma."

I knew she was happy with me. She began to tease me as I ate whatever was left because it would be broccoli or brussel sprouts, the things most children wouldn't eat. She'd say, "Now open up and eat your food."

Then Adrienne's headaches returned and were much worse this time. She even became comatose. Oxygen tubes were placed in her nostrils. Late in the evening on December 17, the operating room staff was called back for emergency surgery. Adrienne was unconscious when she was carried into the operating room this time. Again Jimmie and I sat all night, waiting for news, looking at each other. Sometimes we took turns lying down on the lonely hospital bed, wondering how much trauma a human body could endure. We had no premonition, no sign of encouragement from Heaven, but we knew instinctively this operation was different. And it was.

Dr. Garcia came back to the room about dawn the following morning. I did *not* hear, "Well, we did what we set out to do."

I'm not sure what he said as he talked in his calm unhurried way, telling us Adrienne was in the Intensive Care Unit in a state of constant convulsion. I have no idea what he said happened or what went wrong, but Jimmie and I went right down to her bed.

Adrienne's bed was in the far corner of the six-bed Intensive Care Unit, and she was "out of it." I cannot say coma; I am unable to say she didn't know what was going on — she was just "out of it."

I touched her, kissed her, and after a few moments, we were asked to leave. There were visiting times every hour on the hour for five minutes. No order from anyone could change that.

Jimmie and I walked down the stairs, and there on the landing as the sun came up, we hung on to each other for the first time and wept uncontrollably.

All of a sudden, I realized Jimmie was crying, and I began to get myself together to try to help him. Adrienne couldn't use me in any way right now, but he could. After a time, we walked outside to the neutral ground on Jefferson Davis Parkway in front of the hospital. There we walked up and down. I have never seen a human being suffer such mental anguish and sorrow for another as I watched Jimmie that day.

I, too, was so distraught; I didn't know what to do to help; and, certainly there was nothing to say. I assured myself that just walking arm in arm with him was the best I could offer.

As we walked, I saw something else happen to Jimmie. Before he had been struggling with his feelings toward God. His relationship with God had cooled by all that had happened to our children, but that day Jimmie had had his fill. He was incapable of nourishing his faith in God any longer. I don't feel Jimmie lost his faith because that is a gift from God. But when one doesn't work at keeping that faith alive, it might as well be lost. After walking for some time, Jimmie remarked, "It's a marvel this neutral ground doesn't sink with all the tears I've dropped on it today."

Jimmie and I did go in to see Adrienne every hour on the hour all day for five minute periods, but there were still fifty-five minutes to spend on either side of that five. I don't know how we filled those minutes, but the next on the hour always arrived, so obviously we did something. We decided not to go every hour during the night because we considered our rest important, not knowing what might be demanded of us.

Our friend, Father Philip Hornung, did something that first night that was far beyond the call of duty. He talked the nurses into letting him spend the night in ICU with Adrienne, who knew him well. When we learned of this the next morning, I was so overcome by his willingness to do that for Adrienne that I don't believe there was an adequate thank you possible. I just hoped God would make Father Hornung aware of what a tremendous deed he had done.

By evening of the next day, Adrienne's convulsions were subsiding. Her body began to relax. When this happened, Dr. Garcia ordered her brought back to us in her hospital room. We could talk to her when she had a few lucid minutes. As soon as she became irritated, she was sedated. Dr. Garcia gave me the authority to order the sedative. During those waking times, Jimmie and I realized Adrienne was unable to see very well. Her vision had been severely impaired.

Jimmie and I stood anxiously by Adrienne's bed when the sedation wore off and gave her liquids as well as other nourishment to keep up her strength. With every odd against her, we could see Adrienne struggling to be her old self each time she was lucid. She asked for books again, but this time she only put them aside because she couldn't read the print. I believe she didn't know she couldn't see. When she picked up the book, she seemed to be thinking, *Well, I don't want to read after all.* She never said, "I can't see!"

After Dr. Garcia performed tests, the fact that her vision was affected became obvious even to her. Now she asked for her records and record player. As usual, anything she wanted, she got.

Jimmie had to go back to work, but I stayed on, never leaving Adrienne's hospital room for any reason. I left the bathroom door open and talked in running conversation as I brushed my teeth and bathed myself in the sink. I slept on a cot right beside her bed, never making a sound. When she was able to sleep, I guarded her from all disturbances. I didn't let anyone into the room when she was sedated so she'd have complete rest.

On December 21, only three days later, Adrienne's shunt began malfunctioning again. There seemed to be no end to the surgery and suffering. The decision for this surgical procedure was made suddenly, and Adrienne returned to surgery to have a flushing device implanted on the lower part of the ventriculo-peritoneal shunt.

Jimmie arrived right after Adrienne had been taken into the operating room. Once again, he told me, "There's nothing we can do for about an hour. We should go to the toy store and buy other presents for Santa Claus to give her because all the ones we have are designed for children with normal sight."

Knowing how uncertain our free time would be around Christmas, I'd shopped early and already had all Adrienne's gifts. Those surprises had been chosen for her very carefully— a doll with long hair and a trunk filled with a wardrobe for all seasons, shoes, dresses, and hairpieces for every doll outfit, even ice skates for the winter. All these exquisite pieces would have to be relegated to a closet shelf, and new choices would now have to be made.

Jimmie and I hurried to the Toy Center and looked for all the toys that made sounds. This was an extremely emotional experience for both of us, but we chose carefully because we wanted so much to give Adrienne some kind of joy on Christmas, knowing there was no way she would be at home for December 25.

During all these episodes, we had to leave our other three children to be with Adrienne in the hospital. I insisted our three children stay at home with my regular household servants. I don't know exactly why I found consolation in their being at home, keeping the same daily routine. I didn't want them spread out in different homes with family and friends. That decision might have been selfish on my part, but I believed a routine was advantageous for them. Their lives were actually less disturbed by their staying in the same surroundings doing the same things they did when I was around. If they were packed up and taken somewhere different each time, they'd have felt our absence all the more keenly. Anyway, Jimmie was always there at night unless Adrienne was experiencing surgery during the night.

Christmas was only three days away. Most of the time, Adrienne was asleep because of the powerful sedation. Dr. Garcia wanted her brain relaxed. Since the human body has such strong recuperative powers, he hoped her brain cells would rebuild with proper time and rest. Jimmie and I decided I'd spend Christmas Eve night at home and play Santa Claus for our other three children while Jimmie spent Christmas Eve with Adrienne. On Christmas Day he'd return to Thibodaux, and I'd spend the day with Adrienne.

The anticipation of Santa Claus on Christmas morning aroused everyone by five in the morning. I can't deny I had a great time seeing Jeanne, Robert and David enjoy their gifts.

I left by 6:30 AM to relieve Jimmie. He was to wait for me in Adrienne's hospital room, but she was so deeply sedated early that morning that he asked a nurse to watch her until I arrived.

Jimmie and I met as our paths crossed near the Mississippi River Bridge. We pulled over on the side of the road, and there on the neutral ground, we kissed to wish each other a Merry Christmas. That was how Jimmie and I spent Christmas Day — out on Highway 90.

This was the worst Christmas we ever had. Jimmie had fire in his eyes as he said, "If we ever live through this, I promise you we're going to concentrate on our happiness. We're going to travel the world over, and we're going to have fun." In time, he would fulfill his promise.

Jimmie returned to Thibodaux where he and our children spent Christmas with his family. All the commotion there helped him forget about the heartache in New Orleans, at least temporarily.

I was happy during my day because I was with Adrienne. I knew that was where God wanted me to be. She lay in a deep sleep, not knowing it was Christmas. During those sedated times, her body had a gray color as she breathed with shallow breaths. I kept the room shaded not to disturb her and rocked in the dark until the day finally ended. Adrienne never knew it was Christmas. She didn't open any of the second set of presents we had carefully selected for her.

Gradually, after many long days and nights, she began to have a few waking hours. She didn't sit up very well alone because she was now visibly weak. As a diversion each day, I took her down the hall to a bathroom with a tub, picked her up and bathed her while holding her in my arms in the tub as we bathed together. The water seemed to relax her, and the change in scenery was welcome, although it was only a dark room with a tub.

While Adrienne slept under sedation, I sometimes watched TV, using an earplug to help pass the long hours and being sure no sound from the TV disturbed her when she needed rest.

Chapter Twenty-Seven

And So It Ends

*H*ours and days turned into weeks and slowly crept by. Dr. Garcia finally let us go home. St. Joseph Hospital in Thibodaux loaned us a hospital bed and a child's wheelchair. We made Adrienne as comfortable as possible under the circumstances.

But a new problem began to surface. Jimmie had to give Adrienne digitalis daily by using a hypodermic needle. At the site of each injection, she developed fat necrosis as the fatty cells on her buttocks began to die off. The necrosis created little areas of depression, and her little rear became like the surface of the moon. Less and less area became available to combat the heart failure with those digitalis injections.

Adrienne was awake and alert a few hours each day. So I wrote the School for the Blind in Baton Rouge to request special records of children's books. Adrienne listened, but never with much interest. At least we made an attempt to pacify her.

One afternoon she said, "I'm lonesome for Bret and Mark. I want them to come to see me!"

I didn't know them or their families, but I called a few people and located Brett and Mark. I introduced myself over the phone to their mothers and explained how much it would mean to us to have Brett and Mark come for an hour or so to visit with Adrienne.

I've never seen two better-mannered young boys. They immediately spotted the barn and outdoor playground equipment in the backyard. Knowing little boys, I saw by their expressions that they'd like to play outside. However, they came in and sat by Adrienne's bed until she fell asleep. Then they asked if they could go outside until she awakened, but also asked if I'd call them as soon as Adrienne wanted to talk again. Adrienne had renewed her friendships with her classmates.

*****

Because Jimmie felt I needed some time during the twenty-four hours to take care of myself, to grocery shop, and to be with the other children, we hired a practical nurse. This nurse was the first person I'd ever seen Adrienne not like. But it wasn't the person she disliked, Adrienne soon learned that when the nurse was on duty, we'd be in the other part of the house. However, the nurse's duty was to simply sit with Adrienne and watch her while she slept. When Adrienne was awake, she wanted us. Adrienne had developed a physical insecurity for us.

Dr. Hansen, our pediatrician, came out to the house each day to check on Adrienne. He was the epitome of dedication and had a great rapport with her. Of course, that was because her daddy was giving her all the injections. On Dr. Hansen's day off, his partner, Dr. Mike Smith, never failed to come.

*****

Right under the skin above her rib cage where the flushing device had been placed, Adrienne's skin opened, oozing fluid. We had to carefully watch that area, apply a germ-killing ointment often and cover it with a bandage. This didn't seem to bother Adrienne at all.

Again, I bathed her in my arms in the tub with me, and she seemed to look forward to those baths.

One night, Adrienne experienced a siege of small convulsions. Dr. Hansen, as well as our family doctor, came to care for her. They sat with us for hours until she became quiet again. Kindness such as this always uplifted me as I again knew the blessings of a small town.

Gradually, Adrienne became strong enough to get about in her wheelchair. She had become so thin and pale. But even with that magic drug cortisone, she remained thin. Because the cortisone increased her appetite and gave her a sense of well-being, I felt thankful such a medication was available.

One day Jimmie came home announcing he'd been accepted to serve later in the year as a doctor on the good Ship Hope in Ceylon, which is now Sri Lanka. Project Hope is a private organization with headquarters in Washington, D.C. and was in its tenth year in 1968. The organization had a great national visibility because of its huge white ship with the word HOPE emblazoned on its sides. Those letters had a double meaning — the obvious one — and HOPE also stood officially for Healthy Opportunities for People Everywhere.

I think Jimmie wanted an extra measure of fulfillment in his life. The Hope Ship offered him this opportunity. What was particularly appealing to Jimmie was the entire project was devoted to teaching and to providing medical and dental treatment so doctors in underdeveloped countries could be taught to help themselves. Wherever HOPE went, it left a legacy.

Being accepted for Project HOPE was also exciting because Jimmie had never been to Southeast Asia. Ordinarily he'd have bristled with excitement because it was the fulfillment of a long time dream. Instead, he shrugged his shoulders and dejectedly said, "Adrienne will probably be too sick, and I'll probably turn it down."

*****

Adrienne was soon given another name. Even with careful application of emollients, her lips were very dry, and in her nervousness, she pulled at the skin on her lips. Rather than correcting her, we called her "Mademoiselle Pick at the Lips" to remind her not to pick at her lips. She'd stop when we said that, but in a little while, she'd again pull at the skin on her lips as a diversion.

Adrienne wasn't interested in books, dolls, cards, or anything that required vision. She never said, "I cannot see;" she just never asked for the old things again. Music was the only diversion left for her to dwindle away the hours, and she adored her records. Her favorite piece was "Simon Says." When she sang along with her records and followed "Simon Says," some of the old sparkle momentarily showed again in her eyes.

She formed the habit of lifting her arms whenever I walked into the room, almost as though she thought I could hold her and she'd be perfectly well again.

A strange thing began to happen. Adrienne wanted to smell Marksalot markers. She begged for them, and when we gave them to her, she'd hold them close to her nose. I was sure she shouldn't have been doing that, but, of course, sometimes I weakened and let her have her way because it entertained her.

The other peculiar thing was she'd wanted to hold the gas tank cover from the car and smell that. She spent a great deal of time begging us to take her out near the back of the car. That didn't seem right either. But sometimes we just couldn't help ourselves, and we usually acquiesced.

Finally, Adrienne wanted to go to school very badly. Since the teacher insisted she wanted Adrienne to come and assured us she wouldn't interrupt the class, we let her go for one or two hours a day.

Adrienne no longer wanted to write, but she just liked being there. Once the teacher let her sit in her wheelchair in front of the class to direct the class in singing and performing

"Simon Says." The teacher and principal were surprised at how well Adrienne knew the words to all the songs and kept exact time with a small movement of her foot.

July 1 dawned like every other day, our being filled with deep concern for Adrienne. She'd been awake during the night for no specific reason, just that she didn't feel well. I rubbed her back and legs, tried to read to her, but she still felt uncomfortable. I even crawled in the hospital bed to lie close to her, hoping that would satisfy her need. Her stomach was distended, so I tried using the rectal tube as an outlet for the gas since I'd become quite adept with the procedure.

As the afternoon wore on, Adrienne wanted to visit Dottie, Jimmie's cousin who was a nurse. We felt she shouldn't go, so we asked Dottie to come to see Adrienne. Still, Adrienne insisted she wanted to go to Dottie's house. As always, when she wanted something, nothing on earth would appease her. Finally, Dottie said, "If you don't mind, let me just put her in my car and take her over there for a few hours."

We combed Adrienne's hair, and Jimmie carried her to Dottie's car. She was all smiles because she was doing what she wanted to do. We kissed her as she sat on the seat next to Dottie, and we went back inside to wait. In less than twenty minutes, the call came. Adrienne was sick. Dottie said, "I'm taking her to the emergency room. Please meet me there."

In just minutes, we reached the hospital. Adrienne was lying on the emergency room bed in the first cubicle. Dr. Morvant was with her already, trying to give her oxygen. Because she kept pushing the oxygen mask away, I leaned over beside her and said, "Come on, Adrienne. I will breathe it, too. Let's take deep breaths together."

Dr. Powell soon arrived. I could see the doctors beginning to work with her. I don't know what "work with her" means. I hoped no one would see me. I sneaked over and sat in a far corner on a little white stool. Jimmie was standing near the emergency room bed, holding her hand and begging her to breathe the oxygen. Adrienne murmured a few garbled words and took the oxygen. I just hoped no one would ask me to leave the room.

Then I watched as the tallest doctor began to press on Adrienne's chest to attempt to start her arrested heart again. I was shocked to see the resistance this small eight-year-old body offered to a strong man's application of full-pressure fists on her chest. What a peculiar procedure to be observing when an event of such magnitude was taking place in this small room. A monitor was brought in, and Adrienne was connected to it. I can't read those things, but I knew the beats on it were feeble and too far apart.

I began to pray. I was so confused. This time I actually asked God to take Adrienne. She had suffered so much. The end was inevitable for her. I sat there and prayed that if this be His plan, that if for her sake she'd be better off, then let it come soon. Existence in this world was becoming too much for her. I couldn't believe I was actually sitting there praying those words.

Jimmie walked over to me in my secluded corner to say he believed Adrienne was dying, but in a very calm way, he assured me this was for the best as we both went back to hold her hands. Then her pink fingertips turned white, and the pink slowly disappeared up her arms. Suddenly her whole body was white all over. The monitor showed a straight horizontal line.

Then the doctors I'd known so well and came to love so deeply said, "Ann, it's all over."

Somehow I still breathed in and out. We have a way of having to continue living when we wish we, too, could join God at the same time. I thought, *Oh, Adrienne, take me with you. Don't leave me!*

Then I stood beside her, the frail little body I knew so well. After a kiss, I rubbed her jugular vein until all the warmth was gone from her slight little neck. The part of her that was the person I loved had slipped away to be with God. In His mercy, God had taken a child who was sick from the top of her head to the tip of her toes.

I just thought, *Here she is, God. Please take care of her. I give her to You.*

I don't know how long it took for all the warmth to drain away, but suddenly I realized that although Adrienne was not, I was still in the world with people. I had to again do what was expected of me. I remember looking up at everybody standing around and saying, "I'm O.K. Don't worry about me. Just tell me where to go and what to do now."

Jean Murphy, a nurse anesthetist who had assisted with the resuscitation efforts, walked with me out of the emergency room. She reminded me that, ironically, she'd been present at Adrienne's birth and at her death.

When Jimmie and I reached home, I walked back to Adrienne's bed. There was her pillow with the sunken spot still left by the pressure of her head. The world around me was cold and surreal without her presence.

I hated the passing minutes that would now take her farther away from me and from my memory and would take away the warmth of her body from my body.

It's no easy task to tell one's other children of their sister's death. But we couldn't hide from it. There were some tears, but our children understood and accepted it bravely.

I couldn't put into words what danced through my mind. Certainly I had by now known the experience of losing a child, but it was as if Adrienne was the first. One can never become accustomed to death. During her life, she'd been the true hope of our four hydrocephalics. I'd suffered through each step of the illness of our first three children. It was as if those were test runs to prepare me for the fourth. I was older now, had more mature thoughts, yet that also meant I was capable of more mature suffering.

The past three deaths had taught me that Jimmie was my first concern. For a fourth time, I knew he was still my chief concern. I felt more sorrow for him than I did for myself. I truly felt more pity for all the other people grieved by Adrienne's death than for myself. I'd walked so closely with Adrienne that I was happy when she was released from her world of suffering. Her welfare was foremost in my thoughts. I tried to see life in the light of how short our time is here on earth. Now Adrienne was free from pain. Someday, someday, days that would seem interminable would end, and I'd join her. I prayed I'd continue to try to please God in my life so I'd be in Heaven with Adrienne someday.

I dreaded the ritual of her burial — to sit in a chair or stand to the right of the coffin, to shake hands, to smile at people who were kind enough to call and pay their respects. I simply prayed I could again follow the role society gave me.

On the day of Adrienne's funeral, I decided to try not to think of what had really happened. I wanted to store it all away in a box tied neatly with a ribbon to be opened as soon as I could be alone because the treasures in that box were too precious to review in a busy time. I needed a quiet moment to be able to sort through my memories.

Again everyone came—all those wonderful people interrupting their daily jobs and their happiness, coming to show their respect for our sorrow. I was again surprised at the kindness and love friends can have for a fellow being. I'm sure they were tired after coming four times, but they were consoling to Jimmie and me as they flowed through the line.

This time Jeanne, Robert, and David were old enough to be part of the ceremony. I had them stay at the wake as short a time as was possible. I wanted them to see and respect death, but I didn't want to overburden their young minds. I tried to stress that we were being given a big challenge to continue to follow our religion so we could all join Adrienne and be together in Heaven some day.

I wanted to refuse to leave the side of the casket, but I also made myself follow the directions of others. They felt better when they said, "You should have a coke," or "You should go home and eat."

I did whatever they said to do. It was easier than if I

screamed, "No, I don't want to do that!"

I really wished I could have stayed with my baby. Somehow the priest came, and the last prayers were said. Somehow the children each got a flower from somewhere, and somehow we all got to church.

Father Hornung, the priest Adrienne knew so well, said her funeral Mass. Again the Mass of the Angels. Father Hornung said the Mass with love because we were giving God a saint from earth. I almost felt as if I were someone else dressed in my black dress acting a part. However, it finally ended. I wanted this pain over, yet a part of me was in no rush because this was my daughter we were honoring. Honoring her could have gone on forever. I didn't want the rites to end because I knew once they were over, I had to pick up the pieces and start again. I was so tired of starting again and being brave. So weary.

This time I couldn't put my hand on the coffin to push it into church or remove it from church because I had my three children around me. I had to discipline myself to do what I had to do instead of what I wanted to do. But how trivial were these impulses anyway?

By now we had an above-the-ground tomb of our own. We were twenty-eight when Jim died nine years ago. Who would have thought there was a need for a tomb for this young couple? Now we had a crypt. All the bodies of our other children had been transferred here. We could place our fourth child in the fourth wooden coffin in this magnificent piece of mortuary, the standard above-ground tomb in south Louisiana. Our tomb had a black marble door etched with the names and dates that chronicled our life.

We all stood around as the sun shone on July 2 at three o'clock in the afternoon, less than twenty-four hours after Adrienne's death committed her body to the dark. By some miracle, Jeanne, Robert, and David still had their flowers. They placed them at the black marble door after it was closed. It was all over. There is an eerie sound when a casket is pushed into the tomb, grating against granite. Only those who bury their dear ones really hear it. The creaking sound of the door closing is just as distinctive. The door on fourteen years of hydrocephalus was now closed. Now I had only my memories with which to live. I had learned the lesson well —*sometimes God says no!*

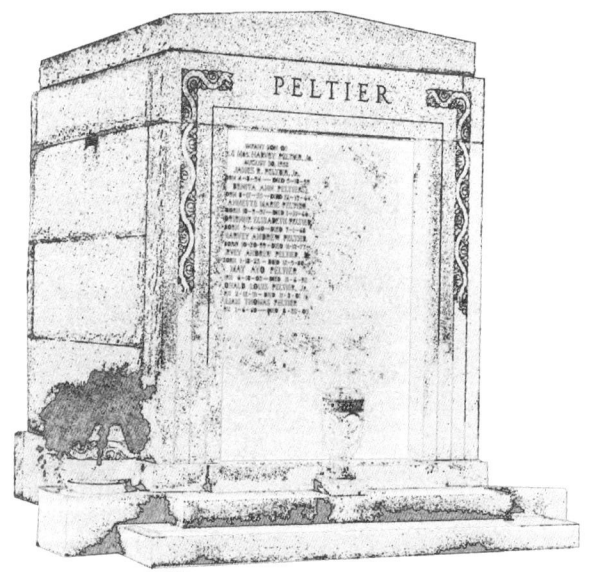

Chapter Twenty-Eight

Epilogue

$\mathcal{I}$ don't know if in a lifetime, people are offered the opportunity to love a person as Jimmie and I loved Jim and Adrienne. (I don't include the names of our other two children because they were so unaware of their world. I don't list Jeanne, Robert or David because they have our love and had other worlds in which to live and love.) From the moment Jimmie and I looked at Jim and Adrienne's strong little bodies until their life was over, I didn't know an intense love such as this could ever be experienced.

We were their whole world. We were the ones to offer the good things — a cool cup of water, a hug, a kiss, birthday parties, visits to Santa Claus, a push in the swing. Most of all, we were the ones who came when they called out in pain night or day. We were the ones who entered the hospital, sat with them day and night, held them close when unpleasant procedures were necessary. We danced around the room to make them laugh, rubbed their legs and their feet to get their minds off the pain in another part of their bodies. We picked them up and rocked them for short comforting minutes, only to find out they weren't so comfortable after all, so we put them back to bed.

They saw us as we were — no glamour, hair and clothes mussed, certainly not offering charming, interesting conversation. Often I think that this is what true love is — forgetting yourself and wanting the other person's happiness and comfort more than anything else in the world.

Neither Jim nor Adrienne was demanding; they were not whining children. We never dragged them to a hospital protesting and crying. They just walked along, holding our hands or having their arms around our necks as we carried them, their faces and eyes looking ahead and observing. They seemed to go with us blindly, yet totally trusting.

That was the hardest part for me. I carried them into terrible situations — necessary situations for their welfare. But certainly not where I would have wanted to take them and not to be carried myself.

Even doctors and nurses didn't frighten them as long as we were present. My God, I could scarcely believe my children's faith in me when I knew I couldn't turn things around for them. I was only a catalyst. No, not a catalyst. A catalyst is a necessary part of an experiment that doesn't undergo change. I didn't remain unchanged except in outward appearance. I was part of a plan, a formula. My part was to be present while all the treatment or horrors occurred.

My mother could always do everything, solve every situation for me, and offer me comfort. With my own sick children, I knew I couldn't "make everything all right." Only God could. I could ask Him; I could do penance; I could make sacrifices, but only God could heal them.

I used to pray and picture myself in the boat with Jesus and his disciples when the sea got rough and the boat began to sink. His disciples awakened Him, worried because the boat was sinking. He admonished them as He calmed the seas, saying, "Oh, ye of little faith." I sometimes thought of myself as hanging to the hem of God's garment, trying to hold on, trying to keep my head above water, and trying to have faith.

We thought, or rather I thought, of taking Adrienne to

Lourdes or some miracle spot to pray for her health, but I knew I didn't have to be in a certain spot to receive this gift from God. I had faith and knew that if it were God's plan and He wanted her cured, it could be done in Thibodaux, Louisiana. But I had learned by now, *sometimes God says no!*

I so wanted Jimmie to get his life straight with God. I have never witnessed so closely such strength of character as Jimmie demonstrates. He and I took care of our children. They came first, but Jimmie saw to it that we squeezed a great deal more out of life in spite of our trouble. It was as if we had to work at crowding everything into each minute we had for ourselves with more enthusiasm than we would have had otherwise. I got caught up in the momentum of his life. I could have been weak and stayed behind, but I loved him. He came first unless our children needed me.

Now I have another cross. Jimmie doesn't feel the same about the Catholic church or about God as he had for so many of the first years of our marriage. Time will just have to pass; the invisible wounds and scars he has may fade with time. I pray they do.

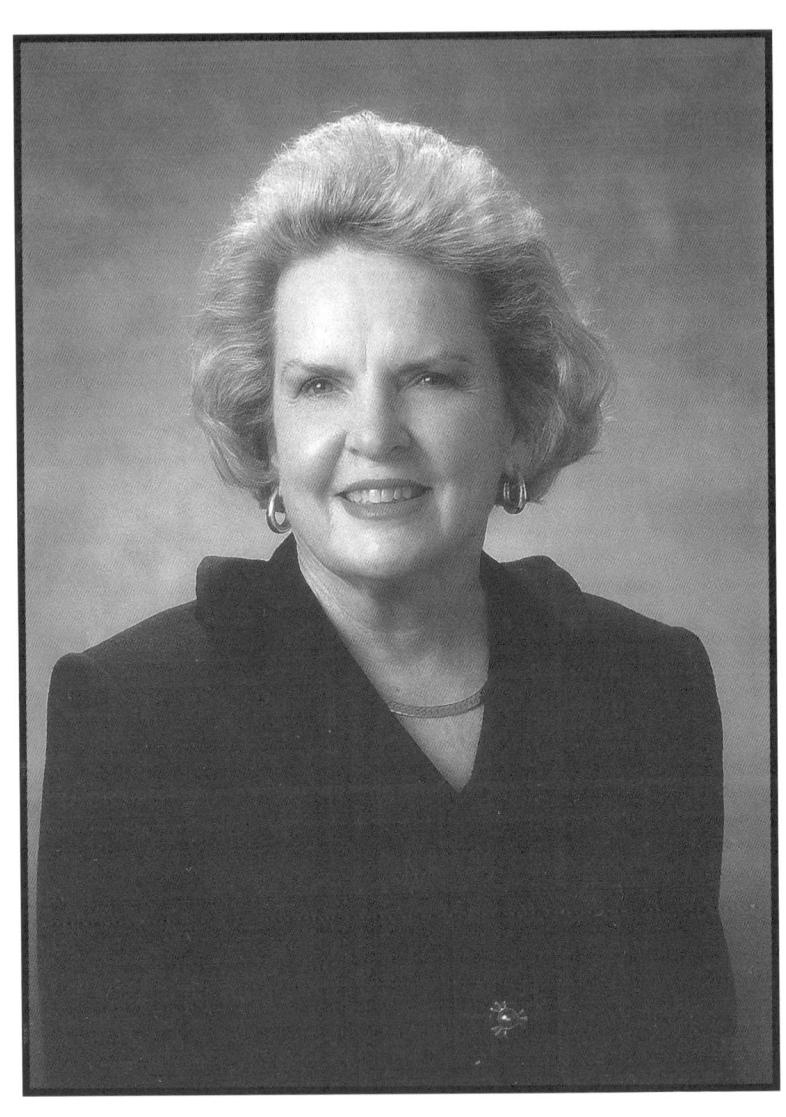

Ann Armstrong Peltier

About The Author

When Ann Armstrong Peltier grew up in DeRidder, Louisiana, little did she realize the life that lay ahead and the critical role she'd play in so many people's lives.

Today Ann lives in Thibodaux, Louisiana, and has just celebrated over fifty years of marriage to her husband, retired oral surgeon Dr. Jimmie Peltier. *Sometimes God Says No* is Ann's story of those 14 years she and Jimmie spent giving birth to, caring for, and burying four of their children born with hydrocephalus. They also have three grown children— Jeanne Ellen Peltier Chiasson, Robert James Peltier, and David Charles Peltier.

Despite the crosses which entered Ann's life, she continues to maintain an active life. Holding a bachelor's degree in dietetics from Louisiana State University, Ann is a member of the founding committee which formed the Chef John Folse Culinary Institute at Nicholls State University in Thibodaux.

Ann Armstrong Peltier remains a community and civic activist and an advocate for reading and public library service. President of the Louisiana State Library Foundation since its inception, Ann is in her twentieth year on the Louisiana State Library Board of Commissioners. For five years, she was also a member of the Lafourche Parish Library Board of Control.

Ann's husband Jimmie has remained true to his promises to her. Ann and Jimmie now travel the world quite extensively and enjoy life with family and friends as much as possible. In between all those travels and that active lifestyle, Ann has found time to record her memories of those 14 years which changed her life and Jimmie's life totally. *Sometimes God Says No* is Ann Armstrong Peltier's legacy to her family and to the world and serves as vivid proof of her deep love and strong faith.